I0094245

THE

TRIAL

OF

STAGE IV

PROSTATE CANCER

JANET M. JONES

A Wife's Case for Faith, Hope, and Help

TTEC PUBLISHING HOUSE
Fort Washington, Maryland

TTEC Publishing House is a subsidiary of
E.Byron Associates, Inc.
P. O. Box 44009, Fort Washington, MD 20744

Library of Congress Cataloging-in-Publication Data
Jones, Janet - 1-1840136141

Cover Design: Noah Urban @mazuzu.com.
Euvon Jones
Cover Photographs: Quentin Jones

ISBN 978-0-9909626-0-1
Library of Congress Control Number 2014957941
Printed in the United States of America

CONTENTS

Dedication

To the Shepherd and Bishop of my soul, Yeshua, Jesus, the Christ, who helped our Uncle Hicky fight a good fight against stage IV prostate cancer. He finished his course, kept the faith, and has received his heavenly mansion and crown of righteousness.

To Euvon, who continues to fight his good fight, and of whom I am so proud.

To our son, Euvon Ryan, for whom we pray the Lord will keep diligent regarding his health.

Foreward

Few people can understand what it's like to give bad news, hour after hour, day after day. I really hate to give bad news, but that's part of the job of being a medical oncologist. It is who I am and what I chose to do.

Whenever I meet a new patient, it's usually a man with widespread prostate cancer because that's my primary specialty. Most often he is accompanied by his wife, and not uncommonly a daughter or son with a notepad. They have usually "Googled" my name to reassure themselves that I have adequate credentials. After getting the facts leading up to their now being in my office, we discuss what it means to have advanced prostate cancer and what the treatment involves. I always try to be optimistic since I know it is highly treatable.

Unfortunately, I also know it is not curable. I try a little humor embracing the quote, "I laugh for fear I might otherwise cry."

Then, it gets serious when we start to discuss treatment options and the, "How long do I have to live?" question. Inevitably, the wife, child, or other close friend asks either, "Why wasn't this caught earlier?" or "What if this had been caught earlier?" I try to walk them past the guilt and the blame so the healing can begin.

The good news is that ninety percent of men respond to hormonal therapy; the bad news is that it has plenty of side effects, and it only works for a few years. That may be okay when you are ninety-five years old, but not when you are sixty. It gives me great joy when the treatment is working, and I am very excited about the many new approved drugs which are making these men live longer.

I also feel great sadness when the cancer does a victory dance, and especially when the options run out. I often say, "Don't worry until I tell you to worry," since I truly believe in the statement, "You're alive every day you're alive...and don't waste that time with worry."

However, it was when a patient who was particularly dear to me came to the end of his journey that I made a special pact with God. I promised not to take credit when treatment works, if I don't have to take the blame when it does not. I can know everything there is to know about treating prostate cancer, but I am powerless to determine who will respond and how long they will respond.

Euvon and his wife, Janet, have chosen to share their journey of Stage IV prostate cancer, one that is ongoing and a road that I, too, am traveling. Needless to say, we have very different vantage points. Euvon was not getting regular health screenings, a recurrent theme among men presented with an advanced disease. I have heard way too many times the phrase, "I felt well; why would I need to see a doctor?" If you aren't seeing a doctor regularly, you don't even know you can screen for prostate cancer, as well as for other cancers.

When confronted with what to me would be obvious signs of ill health, Euvon turned to denial, what oncologists refer to as "not just another river in Egypt." Eventually, when he was too sick to pretend any longer, he sought appropriate medical care. After facing reality, followed by the guilt of what this would do to his family and all the people he cared about, he turned to God. His spirituality and faith, and the love of his wife, family, and community have cradled him. He feels truly blessed and happy with how well he again feels, and with joy embraces each and every day.

Whenever I see him at his monthly clinic visits, he always has a big smile, and it always triggers a big smile back. These are the good times.

Euvon and Janet asked me to write this Foreward and to let the words flow. He is not sharing his story because of a happy ending, but as a wake-up call to his fellow men. I have real tears in my eyes as I pen these last words because I know this tale will not have a happy ending. Euvon's cancer is not curable.

Over 200,000 men are diagnosed with prostate cancer in the United States each year, and nearly 30,000 men will die each year from prostate cancer. Some of those who die may have instead been cured had they been screened. So don't be macho and don't be afraid of the dreaded finger-wave; it could save your life.

Janet wanted to chronicle their journey to encourage every man, for the sake of everyone who loves that man, to take an alternate road when it comes to their health. Read their story; then, see a doctor.

Dr. Nancy Dawson
William M. School Professor, Medicine and Oncology
Director, Genitourinary Oncology Program
Lombardi Comprehensive Cancer Center
Georgetown University Hospital

Introduction

This memoir was conceived after my body called an executive board meeting without consulting me first. I was served notice by forces I was not aware of, regarding changes I was not in control of and pain I could not mask, nor exercise and medicate away. I walked around in denial with a limp from hip pain I could not conceal, back pain I tried to ignore, and a loss of appetite I could not rationalize away. There was a loss of energy that defeated my iron will, although I wouldn't admit it.

I had never tolerated my body telling me what to do. But, for the first time, I felt I'd loss control of this great God-gifted physical specimen. I discovered that I had not actually been as good a steward over this temple, this cutting edge fine- tuned muscle car as I'd thought.

Rarely sick, I prepared food how I wanted and ate what I wanted, while secretly laughing at my wife and children who frequently observed organic diets. Worse, I was oblivious to the various cancers, such as breast, lung, brain, and prostate attacking my extended family. I honestly felt invincible, strong enough to function under a regiment of four hours of sleep a night, while spending 110% of my efforts professionally, absorbing mountains of physical and intellectual stress, and why not? I had done it from my twenties through my fifties.

This lifelong unbalanced approach had become an easy trap to fall into, especially when dealing with something I couldn't explain. When I was finally diagnosed with stage four prostate cancer, praying about it didn't seem to be enough. The reality of "faith without works is dead,"spoken of in James 2:20, is a fundamental of God's Word, which I ignored. Therefore, in the midst of this stage IV diagnosis, I still had a responsibility.

To say I was afraid while still trusting God would be an understatement. Being afraid because of the pain and trusting God because of who He is were two realities in a locked duel for attention.

At the height of my feeble attempt to manage the pain, my bones would ache so much, I couldn't get comfortable sitting, lying down, bending over, or standing. My body refused to be regulated, making me feel like a cruise liner was forcing its way through my digestive system.

My worship and prayer life had become very basic at 2:00 or 3:00 in the morning, when I would end up in the bathroom on my hands and knees praying for the painful process of elimination, feeling like Moses praying for the parting of the Red Sea. Sometimes, all I could pray was "God, just take me home."

With all that in mind, my lack of attention to my health has affected the very lives I care about the most; my wife, children, and grandchildren. And since they've been involuntarily forced into this enormous trial with me, I owe it to them to talk about it and to include them in my healing process.

I am thankful for the prolific Georgetown Hospital Lombardi Prostate Cancer team headed by Dr. Nancy Dawson, who meticulously navigates this journey.

On a professional level, I have received unsurmountable support and concern from Hubert Cave, CEO, Champion, Inc.; Mr. Junior Cubbage, master carpenter and builder for Pollard Industries, and Leonard Stover, governor and senior affairs administrator for the Sant Estate, both prostate cancer survivors.

I appreciate the fervent prayers of my family and friends, including my sister, Olivia, and her church family, and my brothers, William, his wife, Ruby, and Sonnie, and his wife, Cathy; my many devoted cousins; Pastors James O'Keefe, Dennis Davenport, Steve Wilburn, Frank Hooker, Bob Probert, John Evans, Tony Brazelton, and John Cherry, Sr.; the From The Heart Intercessory Prayer Team and Prison Ministry, Mother Mary Lee, and Laverne Barrientos.

The constant encouragement from fellow cancer patients, Uncle Hicky and Dean Jones, has humbled me, and my close relationship with my cousin, Quentin Jones, and brother-in-law, Ronald Smith, keeps me energetic and focused.

Our children, Tara, Cristina, T'hai, and E. Ryan, along with our grandchildren, Symone, Jordan, Tylind, and Ryen, have literally been on the front lines praying and providing physical support, locking arms in this battle with me.

My faithful wife has been a student of my diagnosis, a coach over our lifestyle choices, and a cheerleader for my healing according to God's grace, and for that I am especially blessed.

Noah Urban, his mother, Terri, and brothers, Josh and Zakk, have helped guide Janet from pen to print and have been an important part of our lives for many years, along with our other neighbors in our small, close-knit community.

I am also grateful that I don't have to bear or figure this all out alone, as many in this situation have been less fortunate.

So, to honor our families and bodies, Men, GET YOUR REGULAR CHECKUPS! GET YOUR PHYSICAL CHECKUPS! GET YOUR CHECKUPS! Don't wait to hurt before getting your examinations, including but not limited to colonoscopies, blood work, dental work, and other laboratory tests. Whether young or old, get your checkups.

Euvon Jones

The Time I Found Out My Grandfather Had Cancer

It was a summer evening and the whole family was at a restaurant for a family reunion. But it didn't feel like a family reunion because all the grown-ups were outside huddled in a corner talking.

So, I said to the kids, "Let's go outside and play tag." We did, and the person who was "It" was focusing on one person, which was me! So, I hid behind a cement wall and crept over to where the grown-ups were.

That was the whole reason I suggested tag, to be nosey, but when I heard what I heard, I wished I hadn't been listening. I'm glad I was, though, because I hate secrets.

A few hours later, my feet dragged against the concrete, and I slouched as if I was a person without bones.

Then, my mom jogged over to me and said, "Don' freak out, but your grandfather has cancer."

I wanted to stop her in the middle of her sentence and say, "I know my grandfather has cancer."

But I didn't. As I listened to those words, they repeated over and over again in my mind.

After that, I went in the car and cried terribly under my cover, pretending I was asleep. Even a few minutes later when I did fall asleep, I couldn't forget it, even if I tried.

It is hard for me to know that my grandfather could die any day now.

My grandfather is still alive, and I hope he will stay alive until it is his time to go.

Ryen O. Jones
Nine years old

THE

TRIAL

OF

STAGE IV

PROSTATE CANCER

PART ONE

The Trial Of Affliction

Beloved, think it not strange
concerning the trial which is to try you,
as though some strange thing happened
to you: But rejoice, inasmuch as you
are partakers of Christ's sufferings;
that, when His glory shall be revealed,
you may be glad also with exceeding
joy.
1 Pet. 4:12-13

Chapter One

Pain

"Mr. Jones, I have good news and bad news."

The oncologist rested on her stool, perusing Euvon's nervous smile, his uneasiness. She barely noticed me, but that was okay. This wasn't about me. So I looked at him, too. Then, he turned his head left and looked back at me, which caused her eyes to drift towards me, as well, making me feel uncomfortable. So I stared back at her, which seemed to make her uncomfortable. Her eyes finally landed on Euvon again, and he instinctively reciprocated.

Then he blurted, "Great! Do I get the good news first?"

I didn't care which news we got first. The final bottom line was all I wanted. What could have been any worse, anyway, than the previous diagnoses we'd been receiving over the past three months regarding pain from simple deep-knee bends and back stretches? Initially, we thought it was, perhaps, the onset of arthritis; so, there was no need for alarm. After all, I'd been diagnosed with degenerative arthritis years ago, officially earning my "Senior" badge.

Over time, though, Euvon started limping. He never mentioned it; so, when I finally noticed it and brought it to his attention, he attributed it to a body in need of more exercise.

Yet, as it progressively intensified over the next several months, I could see the signs that my proud husband was going to need a doctor. He refused, though, insisting that the nagging discomfort wasn't bad enough for him to take time out of his busy work schedule to be examined. He'd simply increase the course of his exercise, eat healthier, and wait on the Lord.

Yet, Euvon hobbled on through the summer, until we visited some friends during the Fourth of July holiday. That evening, while relaxing in the pool with another couple and a young boy, he suddenly came up with the bright idea that he, at fifty-nine, could beat the youngster in swimming a lap of the pool. The boy was eager to prove him wrong. Bets were made on the dangerous dare and off they splashed, with Euvon edging him to a win.

Feeling sorry for him, he challenged the child to another race and, this time, lost. Now, I was beginning to feel sorry for my husband because he was dared to race again. He squeaked in another victory and jumped out the pool before another challenge could be presented, ready to leave. The holiday was suddenly over.

Thankfully, Euvon had the following day off because he could barely get out of bed. His body hurt, he complained, and I could only laugh.

"Mine would, too, if I'd bet a five-foot-five, ten-year-old child that a six-foot, fifty-nine-year-old senior could beat him swimming the complete lap of a pool three times without drowning from exhaustion. My body would feel like the victim of a whale-thrashing, too. What in the world were you thinking? You're not thirty anymore. You're not that spry. Your knees hurt, you've complained that your back feels like it's cracked into a thousand pieces. What did you expect?" And on and on and on.

Well, Euvon literally dragged himself to work the next day and came home that evening still complaining, deciding he must have pulled his groin. Uh-huh, sounded like a typical case of exacerbated arthritis. When you're not kind to it, it's not kind to you.

For the next couple of weeks, Euvon realized that pain-free movement was more of a struggle than pool-racing with an energetic young boy. He paid closer attention to his body this time, and it landed him in deep thought that,

"God's doing something." His typical jovial demeanor had all of a sudden changed. One night, he lay in bed resting his head in the palms of his hands, staring into space, as if it held the answer to his internal condition and what he thought God could be doing.

"What do you think He's doing?" I asked, "I mean, we're both struggling with arthritis. We've been praying for healing and trusting Him to do it. Do you think He's finally healing us?" I asked with cautious hope.

"I don't know. Maybe."

"Well, do you think He's opening the door for you to finally retire? I mean, we could buy that winnebago we've talked about all these years and travel around the country selling songs and pies."

"Maybe."

"Do you feel He's doing something with you physically or spiritually?"

Euvon was quiet for a moment, reflective, contemplative. Perhaps, it was the kind of pain he was experiencing, or the age at which it was occurring that made him think about things more seriously. So I waited until he finally answered.

"Both....and I trust Him. I can't put my finger on it, but I still trust Him."

Chapter Two

GOOD DIAGNOSIS

The throb in his groin worsened to the point where Euvon conceded he needed to be examined by my orthopedic surgeon. He was tired of long, painful days and short, restless nights. So, he seemed satisfied with his decision to see the doctor one day on his way home from work.

Euvon returned from his examination that evening happy and relieved.

"It was just like we thought," he said. "The x-rays showed I have arthritis in the hip, and the doctor prescribed ibuprofen for pain, which is good. I can take this without missing work. Piece o' cake."

"But," I wondered, "You said the pain was in your groin and thigh."

"It is, but, he explained that hip arthritis can manifest itself in those areas. He didn't think I needed anything stronger than this extra strength stuff. So, I'm looking forward to getting this pain out of here."

Euvon took his medicine faithfully, and the pain, although still hanging around, gradually dulled. The limp went almost dormant, and he returned to his old self - somewhat.

The ibuprofen had apparently stolen his appetite for dinner, the most important meal to him next to breakfast and lunch. Usually, at the end of his day, he'd dive into a home-cooked meal, savoring every bite. Eating wasn't simply nourishment for him; it was euphoric. And he enjoyed my cooking to the tune of more than fifty pounds since the day we'd married.

Now, though, he'd come home drained from what we blamed on waking up at 3:00 a.m., getting to work before 5:00 a.m., and operating under the influence of the pain medication. He'd make himself as comfortable as possible in his favorite chair and nap, with little desire for food, rationalizing that, "pushing away from the table," would allow him to lose some excess weight and, possibly, help the arthritis. So, I prepared smaller meals to help in the effort, praying that God would bless and heal him.

A mere few weeks later, though, instead of the manifestation of a blessing, what I saw left me in shock. Euvon was moving around in the bedroom at his usual three-o'clock-in-the-morning time, and dropped his hairbrush, which woke me up. Near me stood a man whom I almost didn't recognize. He'd not only lost weight, but he was thinner than when I'd first met him over thirty-five years ago.

"Were you trying to lose that much weight?" I asked as casually as I could.

"What do you mean?" he asked, standing in front of the mirror. Unable to get a clear view in the dim-lit room, he turned on the ceiling light and, wow. My husband was even more gaunt in the light than in the dark, and for the first time, I felt scared.

He studied himself from every conceivable angle and concluded, "Hm-m-m-m, I don't think I wanted to lose this much weight. First, I was too heavy. Now, I look too thin."

Then he paused, looked at his reflection again and said, "Something's going on here."

And, seeing him with a closer eye made me realize something was, indeed, going on. So, by the time he had completed his prescription and prepared for a refill, I suggested he set it aside for a while to see how he felt. Some medicines had a way of hiding symptoms, and a few days free of it would let him know whether he had actually improved. If not, he would have to see the doctor again.

Well, within days, the pain returned with a vengeance, and his limp became more prominent than ever.

His sullen demeanor also reappeared, along with the idea that God was doing something different with us, and our lives were about to change.

We decided it was time for another appointment.

Chapter Three

BAD DIAGNOSIS

Euvon was scheduled for an MRI and a followup visit with the doctor a few days later.

Meanwhile, I scheduled myself for a relaxing evening at Morgan State University's homecoming gala. As an alumna, it had been a few years since I'd been to such an event, and I was excited to get together with some of my close college friends. It just happened to take place on the evening of Euvon's followup visit.

That day, I had nearly finished applying my makeup, satisfied that I'd exfoliated, primed, and concealed at least five years off my age, when the phone rang. He was on the other end.

"Hey, Babe," he said, "can you google multiple myeloma?"

What!?

"Multiple myeloma?.....For what?" My heart stopped at the very name; it sounded so ominous. What does that have to do with arthritis in the hip? And why does he sound so nonchalant?

"The doctor said according to the MRI, I may have multiple myeloma," he explained, "and he's sending me to see this oncologist. He gave me my records, and I'm on my way there now."

"Oncologist!?" I choked. Oncologist. Again, Euvon spoke with no hint of concern. Apparently, he hadn't embraced the gravity of this latest diagnosis. I knew nothing about multiple myeloma per se, but I did know oncology meant cancer. So multiple myeloma had to be some form of that disease.

Oh, God! Jesus! Did my husband have cancer? Oh, God, oh, Jesus! Please help me gather my nerves and find out what's going on. I had suddenly lost my taste for the gala and the reunion with my friends. I could only concentrate on Euvon's words and their impact. What exactly was multiple myeloma, and what was it going to try to do to us, to him?

I ended the phone call and researched everything I could about a disease that seemed to surface out of nowhere. Every article I read seemed worse than the one before, and soon, the computer screen clouded in the midst of my tears. Unbelievable.

THAT DREADED FOE HAD FORCED ITS WAY INTO OUR HOME AND, BARRING A MIRACULOUS HEALING, HAD PREPARED TO TAKE SIEGE BECAUSE THERE WAS NO CURE FOR THIS PARTICULAR KIND!

Multiple myeloma, I read, is some form of cancer of plasma cells, a type of white blood cells present in our bone marrow. They produce a protein called antibodies which help us fight infections. When these cells multiply abnormal numbers of protein in the blood, malignancy results, and its prognosis is poor. That explained Euvon's pain, the fatigue, and weight loss.

I trembled, trying to shake off this devastation, but it clung to me deeper than my makeup, melting into my pores and tangling my thoughts like wet, nappy hair. I felt void of any sense of clarity regarding what this implied for us and any hope for our future.

I slid out of the chair mindlessly and paced through our home, unable to grasp what was happening. How could this possibly be?

Euvon finally opened the door, and I snapped back to normal. Oddly, we both acted like another day had come to an uneventful end. He didn't burst into tears; I didn't rush into his arms; neither of us fell out.

He, veiling the obvious notion that his world had drastically changed, babbled on about his day at work until I couldn't take it anymore.

"So, what did the doctor say?"

"Oh, she's not sure what's going on. Based on what she saw on the MRI, she said it looks like I may have multiple myeloma. So she took some blood and urine samples, and I've got to take more tests next week. I didn't realize I didn't have any good veins. It took her forever to get the blood, and it hurt like crazy….."

"Do you know, or did she explain what multiple myeloma is?" I couldn't help it. I interrupted again. His gift of communicating stretched to the point where he would sometimes speak and talk at the same time; but please, not now.

"Not really," he answered.

"Well, how did you feel when she told you?" I asked.

"I was perplexed," he said, "but not alarmed because I still have no idea what it is. I mean, a lot of my definitive feelings haven't been well thought out because of this pain. I was just trying to stay rational at that point because I was also thinking about my job and all the work I left behind so

I could go to the doctor. So whatever it is, I need to stay positive, keep moving, and trust in the Lord."

"Did you ask her to explain it to you?" I had to keep him focused.

"She may have mentioned that it was some form of cancer, which for a minute, tried to position my brain to assume my demise. But, she was evasive; so, I stayed optimistic.

"Well, I researched it like you asked me to."

He looked at me for the first time since he'd been home. "And?"

I explained everything I had learned and concluded with, "It's not good. There's no cure."

"Golly. Wow." Then he paused. Selah.

After an almost endless ponderous moment, he reasoned, "Well, here's what we're not going to do. We're not going to pick up shovels and start digging my grave because I don't feel like anybody's pulling a string right now and starting the clock ticking towards my life's end.

"So, here's what we are going to do. I looked at the demographics in the doctor's office and the patients packed in her small waiting room, and I've decided that while these additional tests are being done, I'm going to look for another doctor at the hospital where I work."

I agreed. Georgetown University Hospital was world-renowned and quite formidable. It also happened to be one of his largest HVAC clients. He was well known there, and he believed he would be given access to astute and reputable doctors to take good care of him.

And then he added, "Glory be to God. He knows I love Him, and He knows I trust Him. We're going to commit to prayer, and we're going to do what we've got to do, because He can heal me.

"And, you know what?" he continued, "tomorrow we're going to get up and go to Great Falls. I'm going to a real Jewish deli and treat us to a giant Reuben sandwich."

There he stood, convinced that God was able to heal him, and he was going to seal it with a Jewish Reuben sandwich.

Chapter Four

THE GREAT REUBEN

Saturday was bright and sunny, yet we woke up in the fog of a multiple myeloma diagnosis. We were determined, though, to enjoy the day and venture to Great Falls, Virginia, in search of a perfect Jewish Reuben sandwich, with pickles and fries. The beauty of the drive through Northern Virginia's scenic route slowly eased our anxiety and strengthened us.

Euvon was familiar with the area's nooks and crannies because his HVAC business was rooted in the Maryland, Virginia, and Washington, D. C. Metropolitan area. Navigating my way through those places, though, especially D.C., had always been daunting, and my GPS device seldom provided any help. It would repeatedly "recalculate the route" before the "warm, chatty female" would suddenly turn cold and quiet, leaving me frustrated and lost. So this time, I was able to relax and enjoy the ride for a change.

We drove through several shopping centers, until we finally decided on a quaint little carryout off the beaten path. It was tucked away in a wooded community with enough seating to accommodate only about ten people. Euvon ordered his beloved sandwich and sides, excited about his much anticipated cuisine.

We relaxed at a table for two, sniffing the mouthwatering scents of the kitchen, and exchanging small talk when suddenly, he grabbed the table and winced, as if bracing himself against a head-on collision. Pain I couldn't see; pain he could't hide had shot through him like a bullet, squeezing his eyes shut, gritting his teeth, and locking his jaws. He struggled to stand, leaning on the little round, wobbly table for help.

"What's wrong?" It was all I could ask.

"I don't know," he answered between his teeth. "I feel like I just got shot. Maybe I moved the wrong way. I've got to go outside and get some air."

Outdoors, though, proved no better than inside, and the throbbing continued. Realizing he wasn't going to get comfortable, yet embarrassed because he couldn't hide his pain, he tiptoed across the parking lot to our car and leaned on its trunk, unable to get inside, shaking his head in disbelief.

I followed him, repeating, "Where's the pain?" I was choking inside, praying, "Okay, Abba, please, not now. We're almost two hours from home, and there's no way he can drive. He doesn't want to go to the hospital; he just wants to get home. Please, take away the pain, Father, PLEASE, take away the pain."

Euvon could barely manage to answer, "My back."

So I hurried back into the deli and grabbed our order, while he tried as best as he could to settle into the passenger seat. I jumped in the car, backed out of the parking lot, and drove off as fast as I could, while between moans, he mumbled directions down the winding road to the main highway.

Then, just before we merged into traffic, he yelled, threw off his seat belt, and tried to grab his back, while all I could do was try not to panic. I couldn't speed. I couldn't rush. I had to focus on how to drive home without causing him more pain, or equally catastrophic, smashing into a moving vehicle.

Every outburst from this severe breakthrough pain sounded without warning. My heart pounded, and without him even noticing, tears involuntarily fell down my face. We were still barely halfway home. I felt helpless. He was helpless. Our spacey Chrysler 300 wasn't equipped to handle the periodic spasms. He was as miserable sitting upright as he was reclining. It was like driving through a murky hell to get home.

I could barely see the road, nor could I let him see me cry. I didn't want him to feel that I thought it was as bad as he was communicating to me in his own way. And he didn't seem to want me to think it was as bad as, perhaps, it truly was because during the short intervals when the pain would subside, he would pant, "I'm okay, I'm okay."

I wanted to believe what he believed. I desired to trust as much as he that the God we'd loved for so many years would see our tears, hear our hearts, and heal him. But, throughout the long journey, not a word from Heaven. Our faith, however, tried to trust in His presence.

Finally, the last ten miles down the highway south. Left at the traffic light. Right at the third street. Left into the driveway. Home.

Chapter Five

THE FINAL DIAGNOSIS

"The good news, Mr. Jones," the oncologist continued, "is that your protein levels are fine, which means you don't have multiple myeloma."

"Great!" Euvon cheered a lone shout-out.

But, dismissing that slight positivity, I remained solemn, expecting the imminent grim diagnosis.

"The bad news is we suspect stage IV prostate cancer."

Jesus, help us! That wasn't bad news; it was a death sentence, and a new level of panic and shock crushed the guarded stoicism inside me. Yet I remained firm, searching her face for any sign that she was playing a twisted joke on us.

Then, Euvon asked naively. "How many stages of cancer are there?"

Well, stop the planet, I wanted to push him off. No, he didn't ask that question. Not my mathematical genius; not my business owner, not one of the brightest and smartest men I knew. Apparently, his lack of interest and experience left him void of any knowledge of the intricacies of illness and disease.

The doctor looked at me, as I looked at him and then at her, while he smiled and looked at me; so, I looked back at him, along with the doctor.

Then, I took responsibility for the answer and said, "Honey, there aren't any more stages. Stage IV is it."

"The other good thing," she continued, ignoring the sidebar, "is if you have to have it, prostate cancer is one of the best ones to have. It's a slow moving disease, and there are many treatments available besides chemo and radiation.

"Hm-m-m-m, prostate," was all he could focus on.

But, I internalized more thought. "I mean, really? There's a 'good' cancer? I mean, who are we kidding? It sounds akin to 'we're about to engage in a peaceful war.' No such relative. So, seriously?"

The doctor went on to explain that the blood tests had indicated his prostate specific antigen level, or psa, was abnormally high. The normal level is below four. Euvon's psa count was 398, which meant the cancer had probably spread to his bones and lymph nodes. Yikes! That's why he was in such agony a few days ago.

So what now?

A chest, abdomen, and pelvic CT scan, as well as a bone scan were ordered to confirm the diagnosis. She also scheduled him for a biopsy to bring all the tests to a conclusion.

"Is the biopsy that procedure that's going to make me feel like I got stabbed in the back?" he asked in a troubled tone.

She nodded and answered, "But you'll have local anesthesia. It'll only take about forty-five minutes, and you'll be done.

I just couldn't breathe, and my brain clogged. What, in the Precious Name of Jesus, was going on? This could not be happening. I felt weak and defeated. Until now, we had not heard from the Lord, though we prayed continuously. Not even in the middle of the night could we hear Him. But we were forced to gird our loins because Euvon and I had to caucus. Together. Alone. She understood and closed the door behind her.

Our strength felt like it was evaporating like steam from a boiling pot of anguish and confusion; yet, we held each other up. Euvon prayed a brief, "Father, give us Your strength and wisdom to know what to do, in Jesus' Name. Amen."

Prayer had quickly become the centerpiece of our lives. Oh, it had been a constant in our marriage since we'd accepted Jesus Christ as the Redeemer of our sins, and we depended on Him, but not as much as we needed Him now. We'd always been a control-freak couple, used to multitasking with a mastery requiring little outside assistance, except for an occasional plea for direction or cry for help to the Holy Spirit.

Now, though, it seemed as if we had to consult with Him at every twist and turn because our emotions were too out of sorts, constantly trying to overtake us. We couldn't handle this kind of fear and anxiety of not knowing; the anger and hurt, the venturing into an unknown area that was so difficult for us. We were completely humbled and helpless, forced to back away and fully trust Him to give us answers.

So, after a short eternity, we looked at each other and shook our heads simultaneously. No biopsy was going to be performed in this small rural office. Euvon remembered when his dad, in his seventies at the time, had to undergo a biopsy at a well-known hospital, and professed it to still be the worst pain he had ever endured. So, if he was going to have to go through it, it would be done at a hospital in the vanguard of advanced medical technology. Georgetown, then, was where he was going to go.

No sooner had we concluded, the doctor reappeared.

"I'm sorry, Mr. Jones, but you won't be having the biopsy performed here. You'll have to go to the hospital because you'll need to be sedated, and we don't have the equipment here."

Thank you, Abba, Father!!! We'd finally heard from Him. We weren't going to some small community hospital across the road.

"Wow." Euvon sighed. "This is serious." He immersed himself in thought, and then eyed the doctor squarely, and asked, "How much time do I have to live?"

"Well," she dragged out, "I don't like to put a time-frame on life expectancy, but, you can live with this for years. There are more alternatives and clinical trials available, and huge progress has already been made."

"So, I have a chance."

"Um-m-m-m, there's no cure for stage IV of any cancer, but there are therapies to give you greater quality of life."

"Wow." Another sigh, "So what do you think?" he kept pressing, "a year, five, ten?"

"Let's just say your life's been cut significantly short."

In other words, barring a miracle, she was intimating what the prophet Isaiah warned King Hezekiah in Second Kings 20:1. "Set your house in order, for you shall die, and not live."

Chapter Six

YOU'RE OKAY, ARE YOU OKAY?

The possibility of a life cut short. Euvon stuffed his hands into his pockets while we zigzagged through the parking lot towards our car. Then, he cut through the silence, mumbling, "I could use a dirty martini."

I agreed, personally preferring a triple.

Then, he cut himself off with, "Maybe we should ask Jesus first."

"Who?"

"Jesus," he repeated, sinking into the driver's seat, staring at the steering wheel.

"About what, the dirty martini or the cancer?"

He mulled over the question for a few seconds and decided, "You've got a point. I'd better not put any alcohol in my body."

"So, how do you feel?" I'd finally gotten the nerve to ask.

"I don't know, I guess shocked - scared."

He stared down at nothing for a moment, and then, "Man, when she said stage IV cancer, I felt like she had pointed a gun to my face and pulled the trigger, with the bullet advancing out of the chamber in slow motion towards me."

Wow. Little did he know, I felt as if the bullet had ricocheted through him and into my gut.

How could something this complicated and ominous happen to him? Euvon was a man's man, whose career, according to him, was in a man's man's field - construction. As a sheet metal technician, he'd spent the majority of his life handling heavy tools and equipment that had become the hallmark of his physical prowess and mental dexterity. He believed it encompassed the highest form of fitness and exercise, and he had the physique to prove it. Whatever toxins he ingested were flushed out through perspiration and hard work.

His body had never alerted him, then, to get regular checkups, and why should he? He'd always felt healthy and strong. Except for the couple of times when he got hurt, he'd have to be roped, tied down, and dragged to a doctor for a simple examination.

When he upgraded into a more supervisory position, and although he didn't push his body as hard, he still felt great. His responsibility for important contracts, large crews, and extraordinary amounts of money had become one of the focal points of his life and caused more mental stress than anything. So, he didn't obsess himself with anything that wasn't important to him or in front of him. He'd often come home still focused on work, and he'd spend much of his time trying to down-drain his mind. Since his body never hurt, he felt no need to pay attention to it or mess with it.

Euvon, too, loved the Lord with all his heart and soul, and he believed his faith was strong enough to keep him healthy. When he became a Christian, he'd become a Christian. He'd been faithful in his church, faithful in the music ministry, faithful in the prison and missions ministries, and more than faithful in giving.

He wasn't this "perturbed-and-hurt-from-birth-to-dirt" kind of guy. Instead, he was vibrant and carefree. He engaged others easily, and most people saw nothing but the good in him. He was the only one I knew who could talk about the love of Jesus to anyone and get away with it without being accused of self-righteousness or piety. And, he was also the only one I knew who could snore in the midst of a room full of guests, and they'd believe each roar was holy and spiritual.

So, what was the Lord doing? Right then, we didn't know; yet, we believed it was awesome and meaningful, as deep calling unto deep. And another thing was sure. We were being lured into clinging to Him and to each other in a more profound way.

Stage IV prostate cancer wasn't Euvon's struggle alone; it was ours. We'd just gotten sucker-punched with those empty "For better or worse," and "In sickness and in health" promises we'd made to each other at our wedding ceremony. Then, at the height of our expression of love, the "worse" and the "sickness" parts of those vows seemed out of place. But now, here they were, slapping us in the face, and we were going to have to pour oil on our wounds and bruises, and cultivate those vows to fruition.

This dreadful disease also wasn't something we could depend on a doctor alone to fix. No amount of medicine would heal my husband. Oh, it indeed had the capability of extending his life and affording us more time together. But only the Lord could truly heal him and make him whole again. Only He could stop this horror and let us decree with the psalmist in Psalm 118:17, "I will not die but live and declare the works of the Lord."

We finally made it home and rested, resolved that the compass of our lives had suddenly been redirected, and we were about to embark down a path that would forever transform us and the lives of those close to us.

The Trial of Stage IV Prostate Cancer

PART TWO

The Road To Now

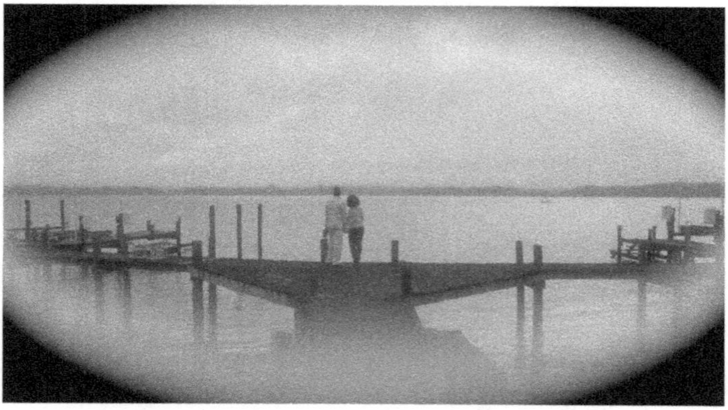

Chapter Seven

REMINISCENT ROAD

Which took me on a stroll down Reminiscent Road, recalling how I'd met this man of mine.

College was the days of new friends, drugs, and figuring out what to do with the rest of my life, not necessarily in that order. Of course, I tried to fit classes in whenever I could.

Singing had been an important part of my life for as long as I could remember, and I wanted to major in it, but Morgan State College required a five-year Vocal Performance program, and I didn't plan to stay one more year past four.

I'd already attended Villa Julie, a private, two-year, all-girl, predominately white college. Having excelled in typing and shorthand in high school, I was offered a stipend to attend this small college and pursue a degree in Legal Secretarial Studies. It was there where I encountered more drugs and racism than typewriters and legalities, and I dropped out during my second year.

Even in the midst of that unsettling time, I had developed a taste for higher academia and decided to give it another try, this time, at a historically black college. So, Morgan became my new collegiate home, and since I also loved writing, I majored in English Literature, studying and analyzing the writings of ancient, as well as contemporary thinkers.

Morgan's marching band and choir had become quite popular by the time I arrived; so, I joined both. I'd also become friends with three other girls in the choir who eventually became my college roommates. Two of them and I formed an a cappella group, named ourselves Les Fleurs, and performed at major campus and community events. Sometimes we were requested to sing at churches and would need a pianist to accompany us.

Charles was one of our fellow choir members and a close friend. His rich baritone matched his brilliance as a pianist, and when we asked him if he would help us, he readily agreed.

Many churches then didn't require salvation in order to sing in the sanctuary. If they did, it was a best kept secret because they never asked us how we felt about the Lord. They only mandated that we rock the congregation and seduce them into throwing chairs and swinging from chandeliers. So, I'd smoke a few joints before the concerts, and then proceed to sing my heart out for God. Charles and the other girls had more respect for the church, but at the time, I just didn't care.

Charles was also a member of an off-campus male band. They had written several songs and were ready to record them when they realized they needed female background vocals to complete the sound. So he called on our group to fill the void.

And that's where I met Euvon, its virtuoso bass player. He was tall and handsome, with an easy smile and silky smooth persona that had long ago labeled him "Groove." He also carried the best marijuana in town, and I was instantly smitten. But, we were both dating other people and were happy in those relationships.

The studio session was a success, and my a cappella group was asked to join the band. We agreed and began performing and writing songs, including one for a popular local television show hosted by a now world renowned celebrity.

My friendship with Smooth Groove soon turned sour, because as soon as he learned I was an English major, he constantly tried to match his grammatical and semantic wit with mine. While he thought it was fun, I found it quite annoying, especially since he'd opted out of even attending college, yet still had the nerve to act like he was one of my English professors, of all things.

I managed to brave his otherwise harmless antics, though, pretty much forgiving him, either when we performed, because he was that good as a bassist, or when I smoked his pot, because it was that good when I smoked it.

Not long after my personal relationship fizzled out, I was injured in a car accident that landed me three weeks in the hospital in traction. On one of those days when I could barely move, in walked Groove. He sat on my bed and kissed me like we had been dating since forever. If I could have, I would have hit him over the head with the traction weight. But as it was, I was trapped between his lips and the weight. And when he professed his love for me, I requested that he please leave. I also asked my mother to bar him from entering my room again. I knew his girlfriend, and I never liked those dangerous games which, in the end, always ended up with everyone losing, except the guy.

Groove, though, was not to be deterred. He waited patiently until I returned home, confined to bed, and then visited me again. While I appreciated his effort, I let him know I would not become involved in a love triangle. He assured me his relationship had ended some time before my accident. I really didn't believe him, and I definitely didn't trust him, but neither did I restrain him from visiting. And he did, almost every day after work.

He forsook those grammatical and semantic verbal games for friendlier conversations, and I eventually found myself enjoying his company. He also spent quite a bit of time with my two-year-daughter, Cristina, who had been born during my junior year at Morgan, and spoke often of his five-year-old daughter, Tara, whom he missed terribly, since she lived with her mother in Texas.

Once my healing progressed enough for me to go out, he took me on the first car ride I'd had in a long time. And in the back seat sat Cristina. When I became strong enough, he asked Cristina and me out to dinner, and we dined at a lovely Italian restaurant.

The more time we spent together, the closer we grew, conceding that we would probably be together indefinitely. And so began our journey as a drug and music loving couple.

Let us consider one another in order to stir up love and good works, not forsaking the assembling of ourselves together, as is the manner of some...
Hebrews 10:24-25

Chapter Eight

CHURCH

We eventually left the group and continued writing together, singing one of our songs at our wedding three years later. Then, we moved to sunny Southern California to pursue a music career, convinced our songs would bring us fame and fortune.

But, not long after we got settled, we had another baby girl, and Euvon ended up having to concentrate on his HVAC trade, which pushed our songs to the back of our shelves in favor of a steady paycheck and raising children.

We also decided to pick up spiritually where we'd left off in our Maryland hometown. That meant finding a black Baptist church similar to the couple we'd attended there, complete with good singing, screeching preaching, and delicious fried chicken and potato salad dinners, finished with a decadent dessert of marijuana, cocaine, and munchies.

We roamed through several California churches until we realized that some of the Baltimore and California Baptist churches were as disparate as East Coast/West Coast football offense.

The Maryland churches we attended were practically identical. The choirs would belt out songs, and the members would be pleaded with to put as much money as they could in the offering plate, you know, to keep the heat on, or to take a meal to one of the sick and shut-ins, or to contribute to one of several building funds. But with meager offerings about the worth of a hamburger and fries, it would have taken almost forty generations just to build an extension onto the existing building.

The good Reverend would finally preach on one or two verses from one of the Saints' Gospels, from a Bible so huge it draped down the sides of the podium, and whose print was so large, one could almost read it from the back of the sanctuary. Too much Bible for a twenty-minute sweat-soaked, swelling, spit-throwing sermon that had little or nothing to do with those two short Saints' Gospel verses, and which almost always ended with a rambunctious, "God is love--hah, thank You Jesus-s-s-hah, J-e-e-sus-hah, yeh-hah, Je-S-U-U-U-SSSSSSA-hah!!!!." And, all in the key of D flat.

The pianist and organist would goad him further, playing Holy Ghost music, driving some of the church people out of their seats, filled with the Holy Ghost, dancing and shouting until some of them would pass out on the floor with broken heels, popped buttons, and shifted wigs. The music would finally simmer down, and those left standing would stagger back to their seats in a daze, sweaty and weary like they'd been smacked around by the all-invisible Holy Ghost.

Then, the good Reverend, a bit worn and tired himself from his own "happy dancing," would extend his weekly invitation. "The doors of the church are open. If there's one out there who wants to be a member, come to the altar now and accept God's love." Confusing to say the least.

The same repeat sinners, who had danced and shouted their way to repeat-repentance the week before and the week before that, along with an occasional new one, would approach the altar to the good Reverend's, "Amen, Amen, and Amen. Do y'all want to become a member?" Heads would nod, and then he would end with another round of "Amen, Amen, Amen. The Auxiliary Board has prepared a fine dinner downstairs. See y'all next week. Amen."

And see them he did. Every Sunday held an encore performance with the same sinners dancing and shouting their way to salvation at the end of the same sermon.

I promised myself the Holy Ghost would never attack me like that; so, I steered clear of all the emotional flailing. I was a spectator, not a congregator.

Chapter Nine

DON'T LET THE LEFT HAND KNOW

The two or three West Coast churches we visited, on the other hand, were sharks after big meat. I mean, half of our paychecks were required to please God. And the pastors brought Scriptures to their defense; not just one or two verses, but whole chapters were devoted to the pertinence of giving tithes, offerings, and alms. They would even throw in a few add-ons for good measure. Yes, God was gracious and merciful, but that didn't apply to non-tithers. If you didn't offer up almost everything you owned, God wasn't going to give you anything. It didn't matter that we were no longer under the Law and Commandments of the Old Testament, we'd better give like the Law required, or else. No blessings. All curses.

Once, we'd heard of a large, popular church in Los Angeles touted as Bible-teaching, and even though we lived sixty miles east of L.A., on a sparse budget and rationed gas, we thought it would be worth it to take the drive and learn about the mysteries of God's Word. So we dressed up our girls, grabbed the last dollar we had in our possession, and drove to church.

No sooner than we sat down, the good Bishop started praising the church tithers, urging them to stand and be applauded. He prayed an anointed prayer, while the pianist played a most anointed song. Then, the tithers paraded to the front of the church like royal peacocks and dropped their riches in royal baskets.

The non-tithers; well, they received no prayer, but instead, got a stern admonishment on the evils of stinginess. The good Bishop announced that if one couldn't give more than a dollar, then just keep it; God couldn't use it and neither could the church. The offering plate was then passed around under the scrutinizing eye of the ushers, who would shoot an annoying look at anyone they thought was trying to rob God. Frustrated with all that tomfoolery, and before the plate reached our row, Euvon put his lone dollar back in his pocket and led us out. The light of West Coast church-going was slowly burning dim.

Chapter Ten

WILL THE REAL CHURCH PLEASE STAND?

Burnt out and churched out, I was forced to step up the role of playing wife and mother. Anxiety had also kicked in because the English degree I'd sacrificed four hard years to earn had nothing to do with washing clothes and dishes, or cooking three meals a day and burping a newborn.

I wanted to concentrate more on our music career and fulfill the reason we'd moved to California in the first place. I would have even been satisfied putting my English and administrative skills to work again until we got on our feet, but I knew too few people and could trust no one with our children. My world had suddenly decreased to the size of a cramped, tattered, fixer-upper we could not afford to repair, one man and two girls; and I could feel my stock value falling.

The ever-optimistic Euvon, though, continued progressing up the sheet metal career ladder. He whistled when he left for work, and a whistle brought him home.

One day while at work, he happened to overhear one of his coworkers listening to a radio sermon rendered by what sounded like a white pastor. At first, he couldn't understand what a black man was doing listening to a white man talk about the things of God; so he approached him about it. The guy was so excited that another brother seemed interested in this young pastor, he invited Euvon to listen to the sermon with him.

He accepted the invitation more out of curiosity than anything else, but the more he listened, the more he enjoyed the teachings about the Scriptures, and it piqued his own desire enough to attend a church service.

So, once again, we dressed our children and ourselves in our church finery, grabbed some spare change, and off we went.

Well, Lord have mercy, we were immediately out of place. I'd never seen so many casually dressed Bible-toting white people fill a sanctuary at such a large church in all my life. Shorts, flip-flops, tee-shirts, sundresses. I was half expecting to see a bikini-clad beauty, or a fresh-off-the-wave surfer floating in at any moment.

This monstrosity was totally against my religion. It seemed like the remnants of the Jesus Movement. We East Coast blacks believed in Jesus, and going to church was a black tie affair. The blacker the tie, the closer we could get to God and one step closer to sliding in the Pearly Gates. Casual dress belonged in the street, not in the church, and certainly not in Heaven.

Then, to worsen everything, Lord have mercy, a curly haired white guy stood at the microphone playing a guitar, singing strange songs to God with the congregation, while they lifted their hands to the ceiling. No hymnal. No organ. No robed choir. No harmony. No stomping. No shouting. That spelled no Holy Ghost. Now, what was that about? What was going on in here?

Finally, another great American tragedy occurred when a boyish-looking white guy, dressed in jeans and a beach shirt, skipped across the stage with a Bible in his hand. Are you kidding me? Not only did he look too young to know anything about the Bible, his was too small.

Then, on the heels of telling a joke or two, the young pastor asked everyone to open their Bibles to a certain Book. And it wasn't Saint Matthew, Saint Mark, Saint Luke, or Saint John. What?! Who was First Samuel, and who knew I needed to bring a Bible to church? For a moment I was embarrassed for not having one. But, then I probably would have been more embarrassed to have had one and unable to locate any Scriptures at all, especially First Samuel.

Euvon was happy and excited, while I dripped with skepticism about what appeared to be a Christian travesty.

The young pastor weaved his personal testimony into the sermon, putting his brief drug life under a public microscope. But when he hinted that he realized smoking marijuana was a sin, I drew the line. What sin? Who dared suggest smoking pot was sin? Why, it was extremely expensive, but it was too much fun to be a sin. Perhaps, it was sinful to smoke West Coast marijuana, but not East Coast herb.

And, for all I knew, East Coast Reverends didn't even smoke dope. If they did, they didn't brag about it being a sin they had to overcome in the pulpit. No, the few I knew about were womanizers and boozers and they didn't talk about that at all. They may have gotten caught and forced to confess and repent before the following Sunday, but it was rare for them to choose to be under the eye of the congregation.

This young whippersnapper was exercising too much liberty in exposing himself as a sinner saved by grace by a

God who humbled Himself enough to take on the form of a Man so He could walk among us, become like us, nail all of our sins to the Cross, and die for us. Then, he said Jesus conquered death and rose from the dead on the third day, walked among over 500 people for over a month after His resurrection, until they witnessed Him ascending into Heaven. The thought of it almost took my breath away.

By then, the young pastor had breathed life into the Bible, catching me off guard. I began to feel as though I was meeting Jesus for the first time and wanted to receive salvation again. Actually, though, I knew deep within that if I got saved, it would've been for the first time. It all of a sudden clicked. I'd assumed, erroneously, for most of my life that when I got baptized at twelve years old, I was immediately saved. But, I never had a clue who Jesus was until I sat in this young, predominately white church, being spiritually fed by a young caucasian pastor with a small Bible.

I was already uncomfortable with the notion that every time I inhaled a joint I was committing a sin and God was watching me, judging me. But when the pastor offered me a chance for redemption simply by coming to the front of the church and saying a "Sinner's Prayer," openly confessing Yeshua as God, our Savior, I wanted to join so many others who were doing so. But pride glued me to my seat and I missed an opportunity to say to Jesus in public that I appreciated all He'd done for me, and it made me sad. Euvon remained still, as well. We never looked at each other because we were both too vain to admit we'd actually believed the wrong message most of our lives.

Yet we secretly, quietly received salvation and quickly became members of the fast-growing church, learning much of the Old and New Testaments. Euvon and I began to hunger for His Word. I especially loved the Old Testament because it told exciting truths of great sinful yet redeemed men and women, and our young pastor graciously paralleled their lives to our current times.

One Sunday, the young pastor invited those who wanted to be baptized to meet at one of the Pacific Ocean beaches where the baptism would take place. Euvon jumped at the chance to finally openly confess Jesus as his Lord and Savior. I wasn't sure it was the right time for me, though, because I was pregnant again; this time with our son. I'd already been bedridden for three months because my body had been trying to miscarry and I didn't want to take the chance. And anyway, getting baptized in a shallow church pool was one thing, but trusting someone to dunk me under the ocean's surface seemed more of a risk than a confession.

Yet, Euvon had such a desire to do it, we packed our girls and a few snacks and drove to the beach.

When we arrived, the praise and worship leader was sitting on a huge rock, singing and playing his guitar softly, while the pastor and several assistant pastors stood knee-deep in water, baptizing new Believers and, perhaps, old Believers who'd finally decided to take the plunge.

Euvon waited at the edge of the water along with several others until one of the assistant pastors motioned for him to come into the water. He then prayed over him and dipped him under. When he emerged, he walked back over to us, excited about his public confession.

Cristina, who by then was eight years old, decided at that moment that she, too, wanted to be baptized; so, we watched her tread over to one of the pastors, who baptized her as well. She was so happy when she returned to us, I suddenly realized that they had had a spiritual encounter I wanted, and I believed if I didn't get baptized then, I wouldn't be sure when I would. So, I asked Euvon to hold onto two-year-old T'hai. I was going to get baptized.

Our young pastor waved his hand for me to come, and when I reached him I told him I was pregnant and to please not let me drown. He just smiled and assured me I would be okay. He asked me if I had accepted Jesus as my Lord and Savior, to which I affirmed. Then, he prayed over me, secured me between his hands and dunked me under. It was over in a flash, but at that moment, I felt closer to Jesus than I ever had before.

Euvon and I continued to dive into His Word like pelicans for fish, eating line upon line, precept upon precept, from Genesis through Revelation, and grew to know the Lord in spirit and in truth.Without realizing it, what once had been close to the same type of superficial, jagged relationship Groove and I endured when we first met, flowed into an intimate spiritual fellowship, and Euvon and I fell in love with the Lord.

We eventually joined our church's praise and worship team, which was a rarity in the early eighties for blacks to lead a predominantly white congregation in praise and worship. But the Church embraced us, becoming a kind of family that while unfamiliar to us at first, encouraged us and charged us with the responsibility of leading God's people into His presence through song. The Lord stretched us beyond our church to sing praise and worship in other churches throughout California, as well as Japan. It ended up becoming one of the most humbling times of our lives.

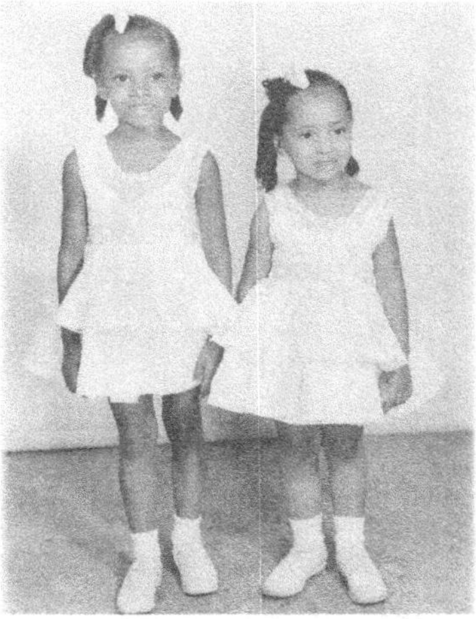

My sister, Linda, and I, 1954

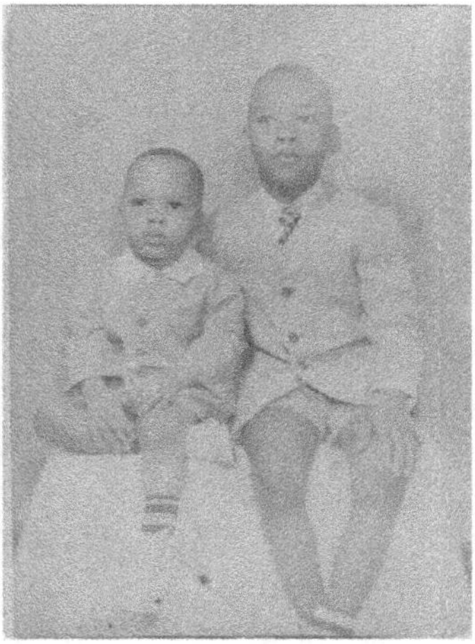

Euvon and his brother, Lawrence, 1955

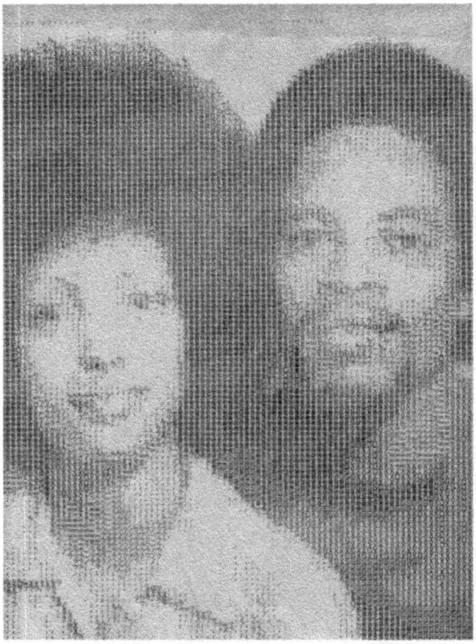

Groove and I, when we fell in love.

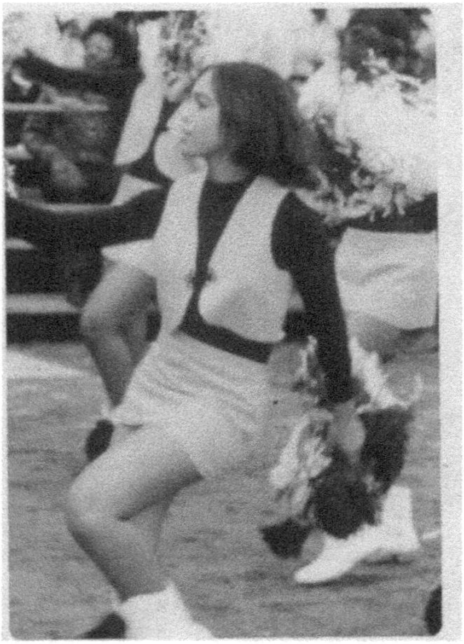

Before I met Euvon, I attended Morgan State College, where I marched with the band....

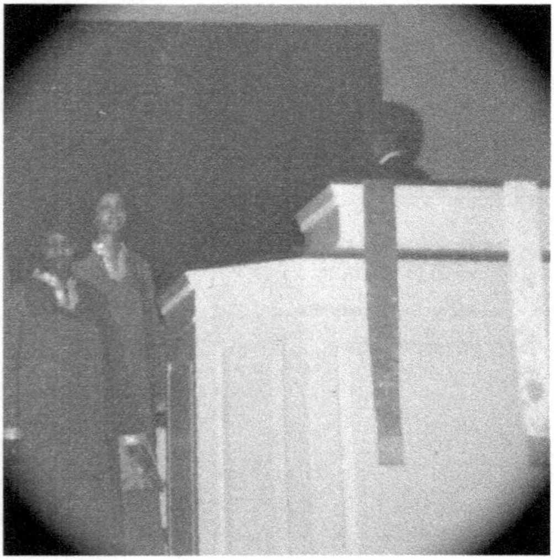

and sang with the choir under the auspices of the late Dr. Nathan Carter.

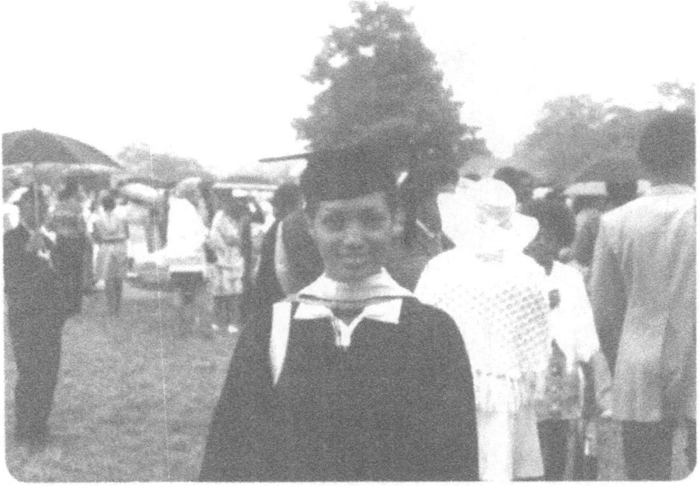

I graduated with a B.A. Degree in English Literature, 1975.

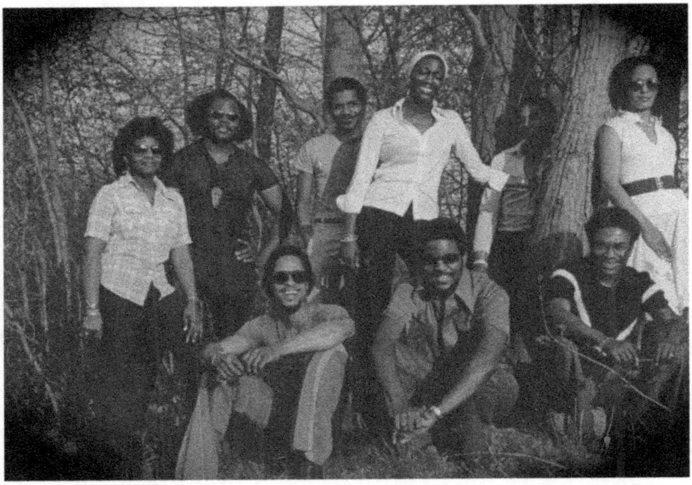

Les Fleurs, an a cappella trio I was a part of during and post college, merged with a band and formed Opus Nuevo, where I first met Groove.

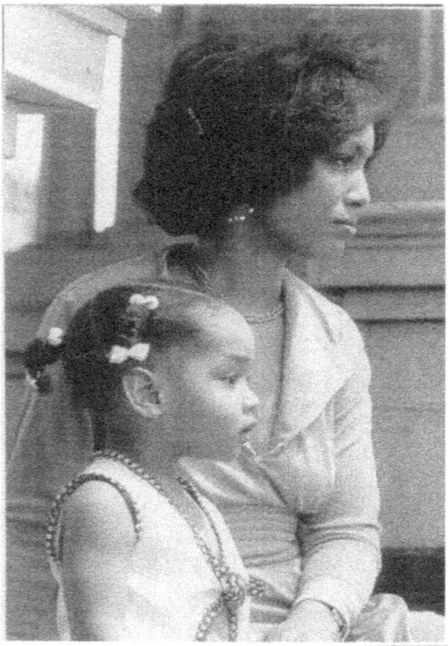

After almost three years of bonding with my daughter, Cristina, and me.....

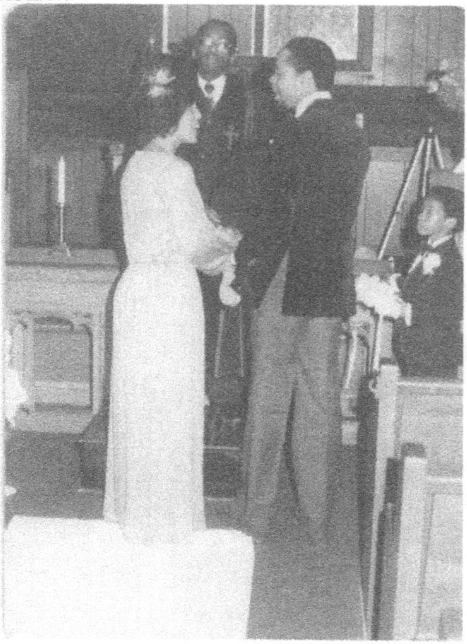

we got married and sang a song we had written to each other. He was now officially, Euvon.

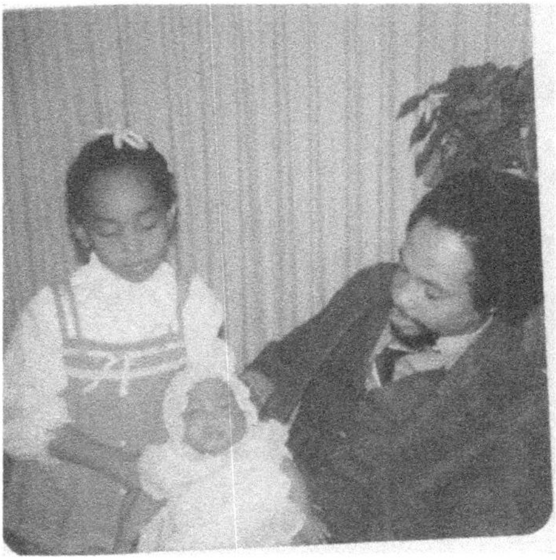

We relocated to California, had another baby girl, Thai, and began searching for a church home.

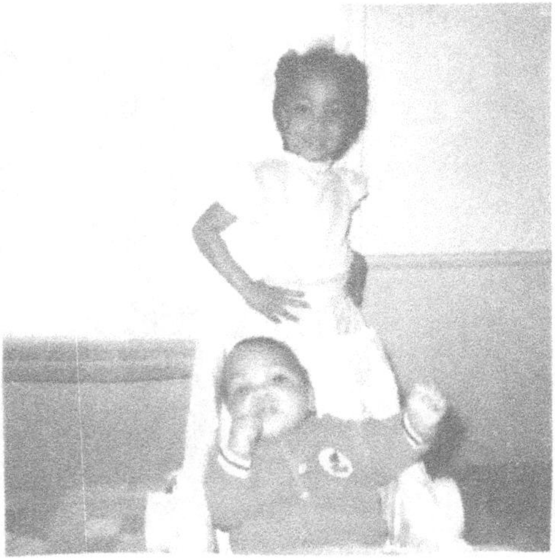

By the time we settled in a church our son, Elvon Ryan, was born...

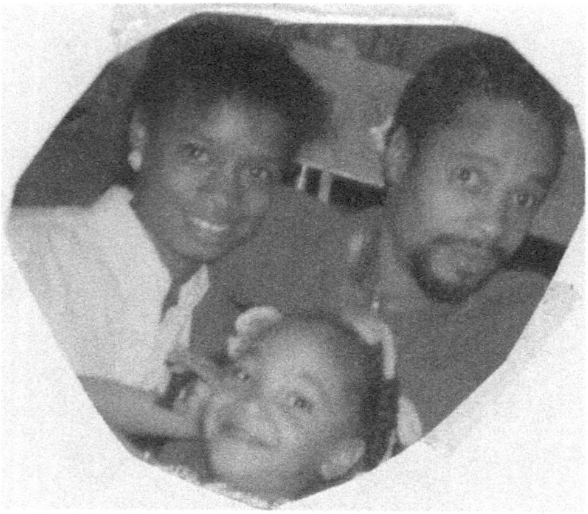

and Euvon's daughter, Tara, was able to visit with us.

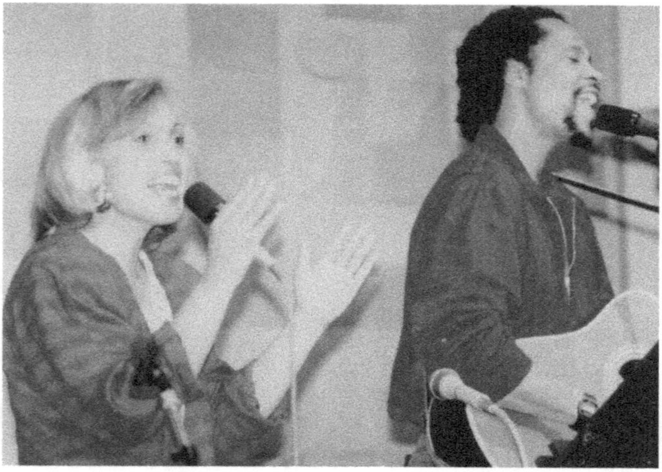

We led praise and worship at our church in Riverside, California...

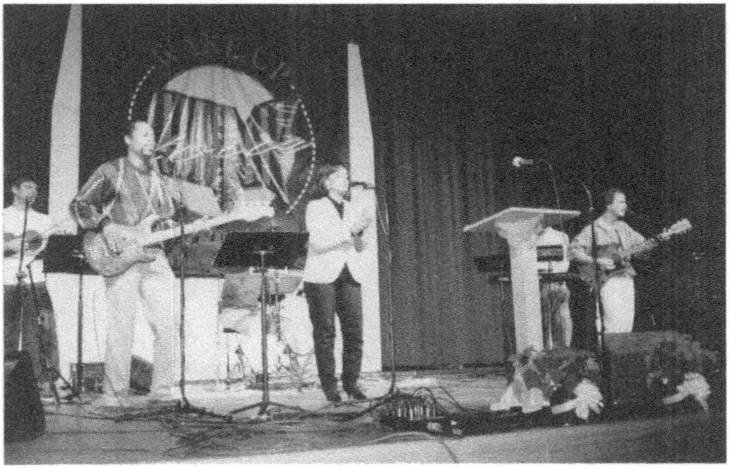

its extended church in Arlington, Virginia, upon our relocation to the East Coast,

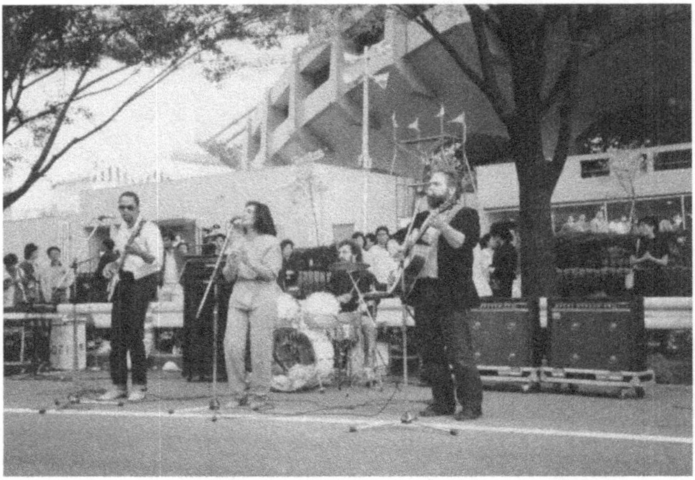

and Tokyo, Japan.

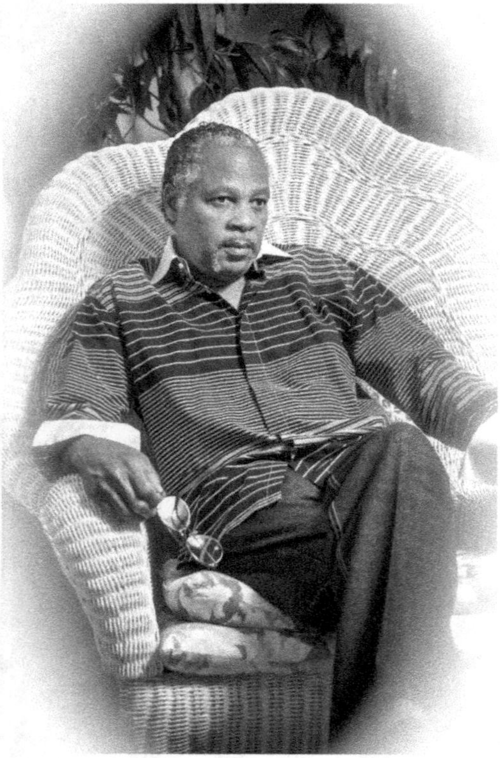

Twenty-five years later, our lives took a drastic turn when Euvon was diagnosed with stage IV prostate cancer; yet we've had tremendous love and support from...

Our beloved children and grandchildren...

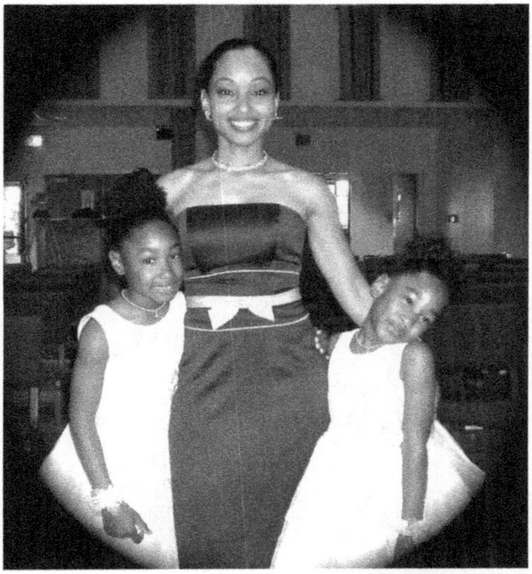

Cristina and her girls, Jordan and Ryen

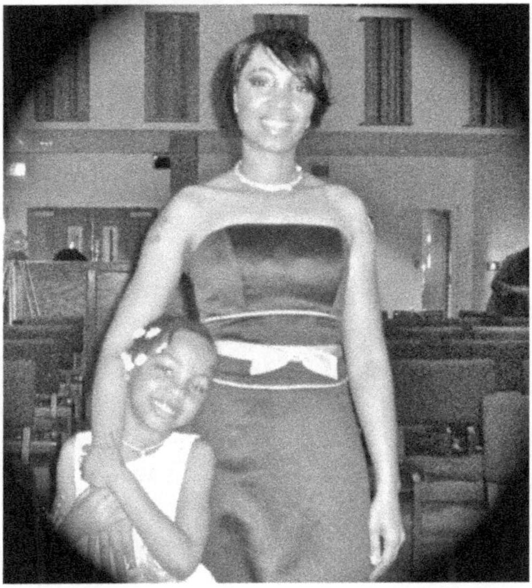

Thai and Tylind

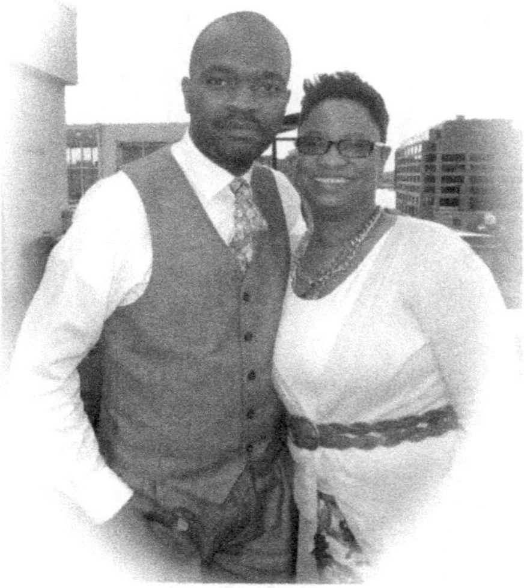

Rodney, Tara...

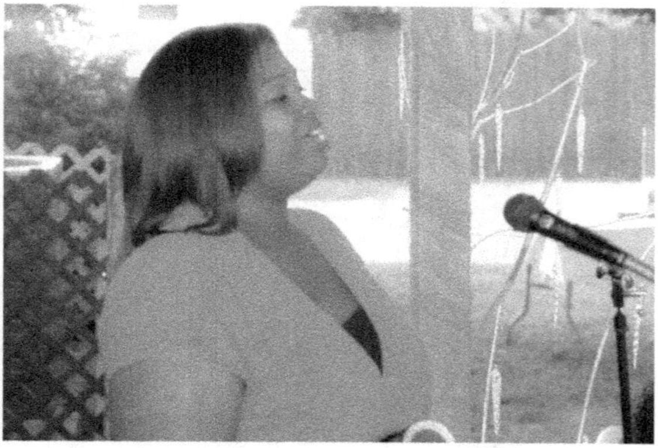

And daughter, Symone

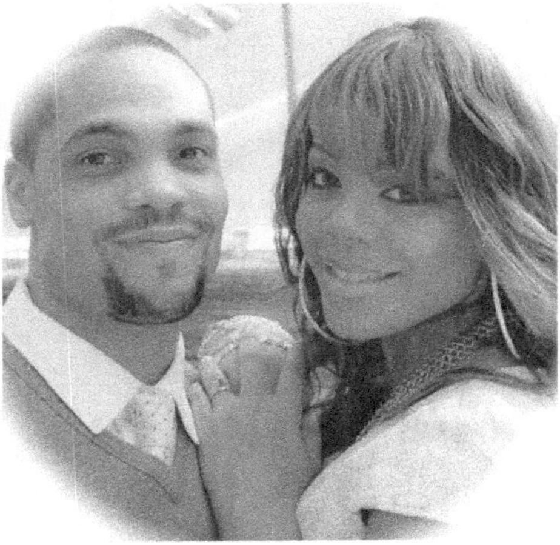

Euvon Ryan and his wife, Nikea

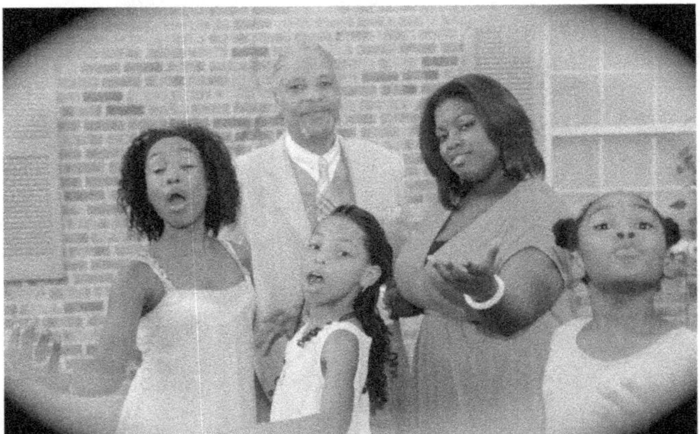

Ah-h-h-h-h-h

and Our Family, including...

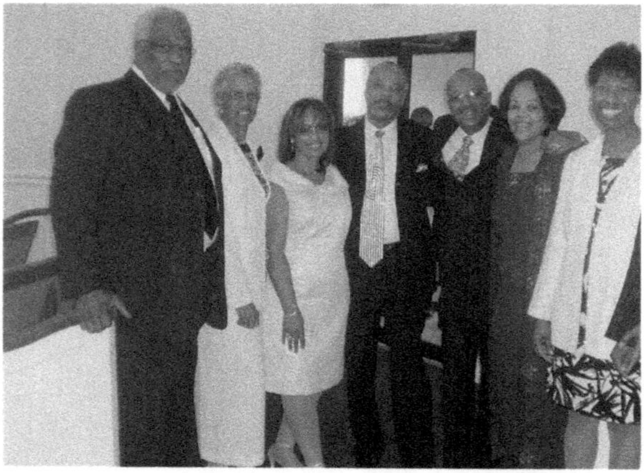

Euvon's brother, William, his wife, Ruby; Frank, his wife, Pam; and sister, Olivia

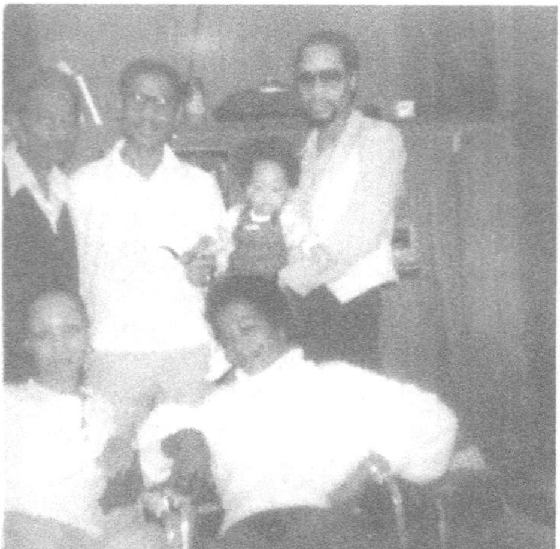

Euvon's brother, Sonnie, late father, William, baby Thai, and Sonnie's wife Cathy

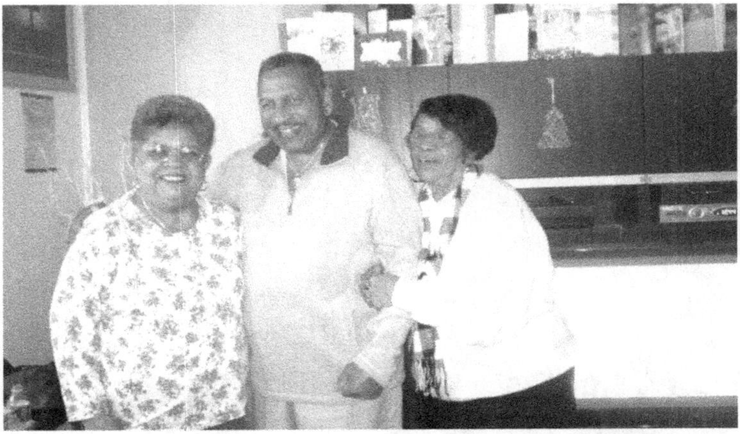

Aunt Geral, Uncle Hicky, and Aunt Jeanie

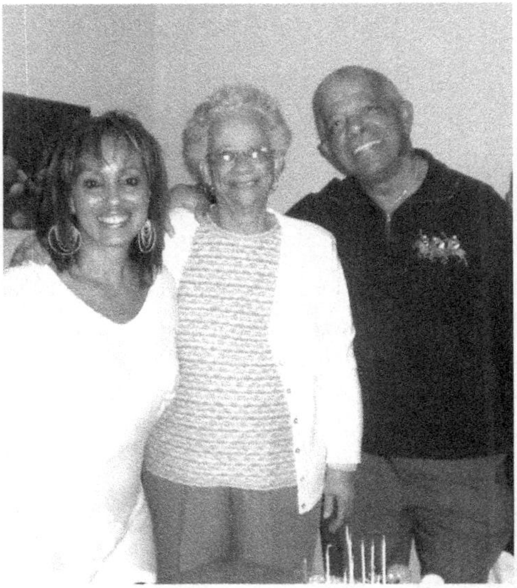

Aunt Frankie and Uncle Zack

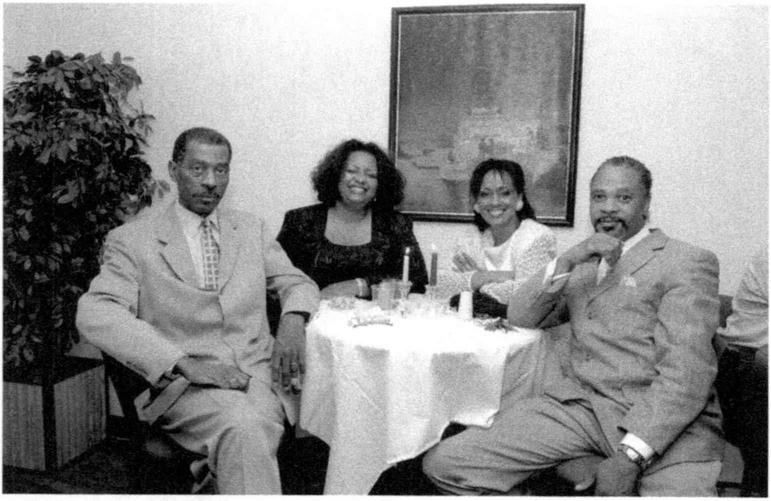

Cousin, Quentin, and his wife, Herberta

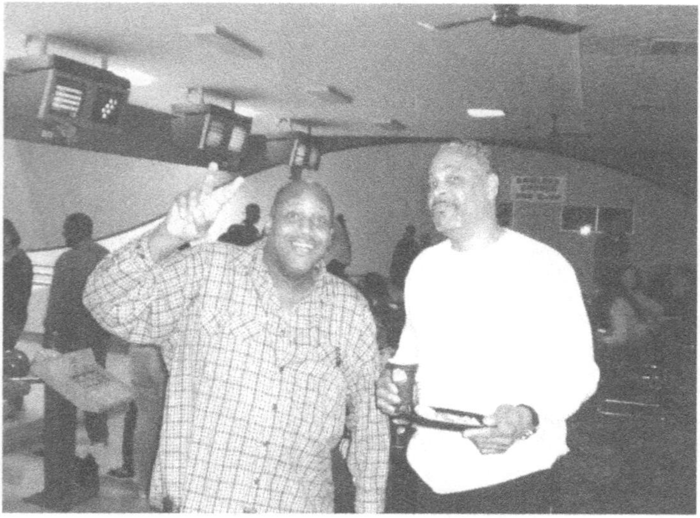

Brother-in-law, Ronald

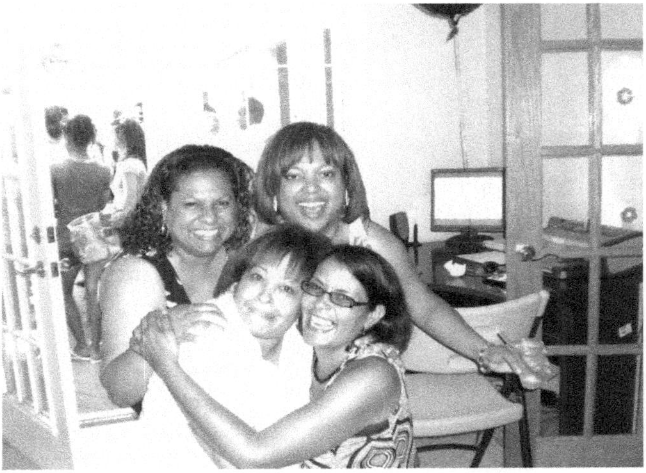

Back: Cousin, Thalia, and sister, Sheila
Front: Cousins, Yolanda and Charmaine

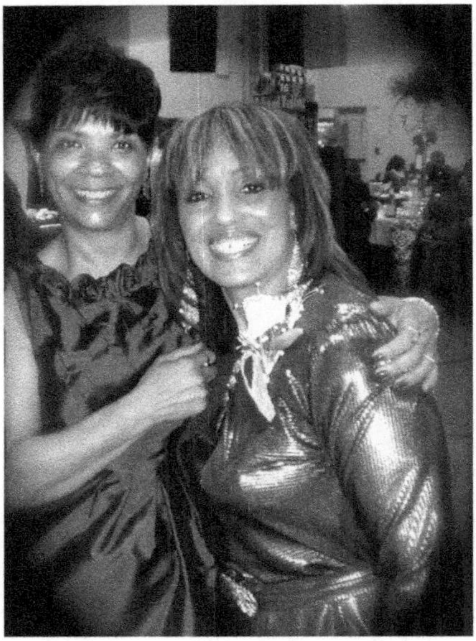

Sister, Marcia

The Trial of Stage IV Prostate Cancer

PART THREE

THE TRIAL OF HOPE

One of my doctors kindly encouraged me to embrace the medical community because while most of us don't believe it has all the answers or know what it's doing, neither do we.

Gain wisdom through research, as well as two or three medical confirmations regarding your diagnosis.   jmj

Chapter Eleven

GEORGETOWN

The towering hospital squeezed itself between several residential neighborhoods, which rendered parking nearly impossible, even as early as seven in the morning. But Euvon knew the facility which had served as one of his most important clients, and that now would serve as one of his most critical caregivers.

He had completed his CT and bone scans a few days earlier and was given a copy of the images. When he brought them home, he handed them to me to look at, since he'd already seen them. I asked him what he thought about them, to which he responded, "I pulled over on the side of the road and cried."

So I was a little apprehensive to view the images myself. But I put on a brave face and pulled them from the envelope. I stared at a skeleton splattered with black patches throughout its torso.When Euvon explained the black areas indicated cancer, I froze with fear at the brutality of its invasion. His entire pelvic area below the navel, from hip bone to hip bone, was black with cancer. Large black cancerous spots colored his thigh bones. From the base of his spine to his mid-spine, black with cancer. His shoulders, black with cancer. His rib cage, black with cancer. Spots in his chest, black with cancer. The center of his chest revealed enlarged lymph nodes. Cancer had settled in many of those lymph nodes and deep in his bones. I suddenly felt overwhelming defeat as my thumb lightly brushed the image of my husband's cancer-riddled body, struggling to retain my brave face.

It was these images that we carried to the hospital for the biopsy team to review before Euvon's procedure. While he was being poked and prodded with needles, I asked him if he was scared.

He confidently smiled and replied, "Absolutely." Yet, in spite of his fear and discomfort, he remained upbeat.

Once he was prepped and ready to be wheeled away, we kissed and waved to each other until he was out of sight. One part of me felt satisfied knowing he was in qualified hands, sedated and pain-free, while the other part felt overwhelmed with this otherworldly anticipation of a death sentence confirmed.

I sat in the waiting room and observed the many patients and their families who were waiting for tests or other medical exams to be done. Then I closed my eyes and prayed Apostle Paul's prayer in Ephesians 3:16-19 that, "we would be strengthened with might through His Spirit in the inner man, that Jesus would dwell in our hearts by faith, and that we, being rooted and grounded in love, would be able to comprehend the breadth and length, and depth and height of His love," a love manifested in a promise in Isaiah 53 stating, "He was wounded for our crimes and crushed because of our sins. He bore our sickness, carried our pain, and by His stripes, we are healed."

I prayed a silent prayer of healing for those around me, for our children and grandchildren's health, and again for my husband's healing.

Before I knew it, my name was called, and I followed the attendant to the recovery room. Euvon was propped against a couple of pillows finishing a sandwich and a banana.

The nurse attending him encouraged him to take his time before moving around until he had regained his strength. But Euvon was anxious to leave and relax with an enjoyable meal. He wanted to go home, and after a couple of hours, while conceding to a little nausea, he was certain he'd be up for the ride.

Well, by the time we drove away from the hospital and into rush-hour traffic, his nausea was in full swing. There was no way with us inching along, that we were going to make it home in time for him to empty himself. So, I pulled over on the side of the road several times so he could hang his head out of the car and regurgitate his sandwich, juice, water, banana, and anything else still lingering around internally. The slower the drive, the more irritable he became, but it was of no consequence. We just had to get comfortable pulling over onto the nearest road shoulder so he could relieve himself.

Once we got home, he longed for a steak, baked potato, and salad to fill his empty stomach but couldn't even retain a cup of broth, toast, or crackers. The anti-nausea medicine he was given didn't help, and after a while, all he wanted to do was just lie still on the sofa alone.

That is, until the pain medicine wore off. Then he had to get up and move, making futile attempts to walk off the pain. He'd take a few steps, lean on the back of the sofa, and cry, "Help me, Jesus!" A few steps later, he'd rest on the kitchen counter and wail, "Lord, have mercy!" Back and forth, back and forth he limped between the living room and kitchen in a fit, unable to cope with the suffering.

I followed him, crying and praying, pleading with God to take away his pain, straining to hear a word or see a sign from Him. "Please don't let him suffer, Father. Please, don't let him go through this. Please, Father, can't You hear us crying for You?"

Then, Euvon's torturous cry for help. "Oh, Lord have mercy!"

Our home had transformed into an Eastern Wailing Wall and throughout the night, he paced and prayed, groaned and prayed. After a long trek back and forth from room to room, I had grown beyond weary. All I wanted to do was fold up in a corner of our bed, hide my head under my pillow, and drown out Euvon's cries. But how dare I ignore his longing for my patience and support or his pleas for forgiveness for disturbing me. So I walked with him when I could and retreated to the covers when I needed to until he finally calmed down and made peace with the pain. He eased himself on the bed and one deep breath ushered him to sleep.

Oh, that the Lord would strengthen him on his sick bed, and in his illness, restore him to health, as Psalm 41:3 promised. I closed my eyes, grateful, with "Praise Him" on my mind.

Yea, though I walk through the valley of
the shadow of death, I will fear no evil,
for You are with me; Your rod and Your
staff, they comfort me.
Psalm 23:4

Chapter Twelve

"I DON'T WANT TO DIE"

We felt rested the next morning, and although Euvon was still in pain, it wasn't as intense as the day before. His doctor had prescribed more effective pain medicine, and he progressed well throughout the day.

Since we hadn't really talked that torturous day before, I seized an opportunity to ask him if he'd remembered anything about the biopsy and why it had caused him so much pain. It had become important to me to encourage Euvon to expose his feelings so he wouldn't drift to a place where I couldn't reach him. I'd been drafted into this war when I married him, and I wanted to understand it so we could march together on the battlefield with like minds.

"Well," he said, "when I saw all the equipment, all I could think about was what they had to do and how far inside of me they had to go since the cancer was in my bones. I lay between my side and stomach so they could go into my hip bone where some of the tumor was and extract a little culture out of my bone marrow. Apparently, this procedure was so critical, I was placed somewhat inside of this reflective CT scanner so they could magnify that part of my body to see where the needle was, and where they had to go in.

"I was only partially comatose, which made it easy to fall asleep, and since they were going into my bone, I didn't want to be awake anyway. At one point, the doctor woke me up and told me they were going to go in one direction but considered it to be a little too risky; so, they decided to go in another way.

"At that point, I prayed because my life was in their hands. They were responsible for how it turned out, and if I would be alive today to talk about it. They could have gone in the wrong way or the needle could have accidentally broken off inside me with the culture dissipating in my body, causing the tumor to spread to places it hadn't yet gone.

"I also thanked God for giving me a team of gifted doctors who were not participating in their first rodeo, so to speak."

Euvon was silent for a few minutes, and then continued.

"Between the day I first got the news about this illness and the biopsy, I didn't run around and say, 'Okay, I'm dying.' With all my faith and my relationship with God, I just could not visualize and get in touch with actually dying.

"I've remained focused on my job and have handled my business like nothing's been wrong. I mean, I've got multiple clients and contracts, and I haven't wanted anything or anyone to suffer because of what I'm personally dealing with. The biggest blessing that's also been a huge obstacle in my life has been that my job has been so over imposing, I haven't spent a lot of time thinking about the logistics of my diagnosis. I mean, I have so much work still ever present, and it needs to be resolved, it needs to be set up, and it needs to be fleshed out so we can address it and keep things moving economically for the company.

"But, then yesterday, when I struggled with the excruciating pain my whole body and bones were going through, it made me wail and cry. The possibility of death finally hit me. When I was on the couch unable to get rid of the pain and not wanting to eat, I just wanted to pray. I needed to get alone with God internally, not just so I could express my own feelings, but I also needed to hear what He had to say. Then, at one point, I said to Him, 'I don't want to die.' I didn't pray it all the time or for the rest of the day and night. Just that one specific time."

Euvon then emphasized our need to pray without ceasing because jumping through hoops and getting this person or that person to try to resolve something about which we know nothing expends our emotions. We'd have to be so on point with the Lord, which wasn't easy because we still had to live with ourselves. Not only would prayer have to be the most important part of our life, but equally crucial was daring to trust Him to help us trust the process.

The Bible says, "In the multitude of counsellors, there is safety (Prov. 11:14), which meant we'd have to listen to his doctors and follow any recommended treatment plan, regardless of its measure of discomfort. We'd also have to glean as much information as possible to try to comprehend the diagnosis and be educated about it so we could pray with knowledge, with conviction, and with absolute understanding of where we were within that revelation.

And then we prayed.

Chapter Thirteen

THE ADVERSARY CALLED CANCER

I followed Euvon's advice and researched everything I could about prostate cancer to understand its causes, symptoms, and management, so that our son and other men could do everything possible to prevent its almost inevitable attack.The prostate is an organ about the size of a walnut but can cause an enormous amount of damage if left unchecked. I was surprised to learn that the majority of men would be diagnosed with it at some point in their lifetime.

If genetics were a factor, as several articles suggested, then Euvon may have inherited the vulnerability from his father, who died with it but, Praise God, not from it, when he was eighty-nine years old. If the high consumption of dairy products, sugar, and broiled and charred meats put certain men at higher risk, as was also suggested, then he was an easy target because we lived on those foods. We would use our charcoal grill to barbecue water because we so loved the taste of charcoaled food.

Although there were subtle early telltale signs that something was amiss, we overlooked them because Euvon had never had a problem urinating, there was no blood in his urine or stool, and the only aches and pains he felt, he thought, resulted either from his work or a lack of exercise.

But after a long, hard thought, we remembered that over the years, he did urinate frequently, another early sign, practically day in and day out. A conversation would often be abruptly interrupted and regular activities dropped like burning charcoal for a jaunt to the bathroom. On the rare occasions we took an out-of-town trip longer than a thirty-minute drive, he would stop at almost every exit for relief, and I could always tell when he was in trouble. He would start rocking and squeezing the steering wheel. Then he'd throw off his seat belt, slamming it against the door, and clapping his knees.

All this time, we'd chalked it up to the thirty-two ounces of coffee and the two or three cans of toxic soda he'd wake up to every day. It never dawned on us that something could be seriously wrong, warranting a checkup.

The first oncologist had informed Euvon that he'd had prostate cancer for a number of years. And because he'd given no attention to any of his body's irregularities, he had already bypassed the first three stages.

Stages I and II, which caused little or no problems, sometimes involved "watchful waiting," meaning the prostate would be examined regularly. Stage III could include surgery, chemotherapy and/or radiation, and a myriad of medicines with possible side effects. Well, Euvon was far beyond all of that at stage IV. On one hand, I was grateful he wouldn't be receiving toxic doses of chemo and radiation, nor would he have any surgeries that could have been difficult to recover from. Yet, on the other hand, regular checkups and early detection could have prevented him from facing this battle at all. Either way, we were in for a dirty, blood bath. Stages I thru III may have required us driving unmarked cars using uzis and machetes to kill the disease; but with stage IV, we were going to need bombs, hand grenades, and tanks.

We spent some time one day reflecting on the good times, as well as the challenges in our marriage. While those good times strengthened our love and commitment, it was the difficulties that built in us indomitable spirits. During our first few years, every squabble ended with each of us raising our fists in our own personal victory. We were both strong-willed and dared not extend an olive branch, as it was a sure sign of defeat. So, we'd remain "victoriously" silent until the conflict was all but forgotten. Then one of us would ask for a lame forgiveness, not because of any wrong doing, but because it was time to move on to other issues of life.

Now, we had to reposition our fists, formerly raised in mock victory against each other to, with one accord, aim at the face of the enemy called cancer, stand firm, and fight.

Chapter Fourteen

THE DEVIL AND THE BIG BLACK "C"

Which brought me to the question; what is cancer, anyway? I'd never heard of anyone catching it, becoming infected with it, or coming down with it. It isn't airborne or something we breathe in, nor is it brought into the body through some strain of bacteria. So where does this fiendish disease come from? What makes it tick? What gives it life? What I found revealed diabolical similarities to the devil.

King David sang in Psalm 139:14 that, "we were fearfully and wonderfully made." Yet, in the midst of this awesome wonder, because of the sinful world we live in, our bodies are susceptible to everyday wear and tear, and can revolt against themselves.

We were created with living cells designed to function together in perfect precision. As with every living being in the earth, when cells become old or sick, they die. When that happens, certain genes signal the process of healthy cells dividing to replace them.

Satan was a heavenly cherub full of wisdom and perfect in beauty (Ezekiel 28:12), who lived in harmony with the rest of the host of heaven.

Sometimes, due to a faulty signal, that old or sick cell in us doesn't die. Instead, it becomes deformed and disorderly, replicating itself faster than the healthy cells, piling on top of each other and forming a tumor.

Likewise, at some eternal point, the devil, whose name was also Lucifer, developed a faulty switch, leaving him angry and jealous of the holiness and glory of God, which derailed his own perfection. So, instead of dying, according to Revelation 12, he influenced one-third of heaven's angels to rebel against the Lord. He had become a tumor.

Now, a tumor can be benign, or harmless. On the other hand, one of its cells may worsen and divide at warped speed, creating more mutations in the process. Then, they infiltrate the healthy cells, preventing them from maintaining their responsibility to sustain a healthy body. They've become malignant cancer.

Well, satan's jealousy and deceit reached a boiling point that compelled him and his cohorts to throw a coup d'etat against the Lord. Another archangel, Michael, assembled his own army, defeated satan and his legion, and threw them out of heaven. Jesus said in Luke 10:18, "I beheld satan as lightning fall from heaven." They had become malignant.

Once the malignancy has developed, if left undetected and untreated, its cells can spread out of control and stalk the rest of the body, destroying other organs, bones, lymph nodes, and tissues. It has metastasized.

The devil and his demons have stalked the earth since before time as we know it, wreaking havoc and destruction; killing, stealing, and destroying - metastasizing.

Malignant tumor cells' inevitable goal is to destroy the body. But, the very thing that tries to kill a person becomes the tool that kills itself. Once they take over the body, there's nothing left to control; so when the body dies, they die as well.

Satan, too, has been dogged in his attempt to destroy everything in his path. But in his relentless pursuit of destruction, he himself will be destroyed.

Cancer and satan, however, are powerless without God's permission, and the devil has no problem challenging his Nemesis for that power to destroy each and every one of us, as exampled in the Book of Job.

Job was wealthy and righteous, blessed with a wife, many children, and an abundance of land, cattle, and servants. He loved the Lord and was deeply loved by Him. Their relationship was so close that satan, in his jealousy, attempted to turn Job against God. According to Job 1, "The sons of God came to present themselves before the Lord and satan came also."

Now, with all the hell that evicted demon had been raising against God since time eternal, he was still given access into His presence. And although we've been given the same access, we shy away. The apostle Paul encourages us in Hebrews 4:16 to "Come boldly to the throne of grace that we may obtain mercy and find grace to help in the time of need."

Satan takes advantage of that verse and uses it today as his ticket to approach Father day and night to accuse us for every minuscule thing we do. Yet, many of us rarely go before the Lord for anything because we're either too afraid, too arrogant, or just plain apathetic.

Well, satan wanted Job to turn against God and so challenged Him to let him destroy almost everything the righteous man owned, including his children. Then he said Job would curse God to His face. Lo and behold, Father granted him his request and allowed him to do as he asked. Yet, in his grief, Job refused to curse God. "Yea, though He slay me," he cried, "yet will I trust Him."

Chapter two detailed a second challenge the dastardly devil directed towards the Lord, since his previous one had failed. This time, he wanted to attack Job's flesh and bone. He was sure, then, that Mr. Righteous would curse God to His face. And guess what? God granted him permission again.

Poor Job was covered from head to toe with boils that tormented him, giving him no rest for his soul. In his misery, though, he poured out his heart before God, even if it was through complaints and questions. But there were other times, even in his darkest moments where he affirmed that his "Redeemer lives and in the end, He would stand upon the earth." It was also declared in Job 22:27-28, "You will make your prayer unto Him, and He will hear you..., you will also declare a thing, and it will be established for you, so light will shine on your ways."

Somehow, in the midst of his trial and tribulation, he found a way to remain faithful to God and to sometimes praise Him. In the end, he found favor in God's eyes because of his faithfulness and sometimes praise, and he prospered more in his latter years than in his former.

Praise God, Euvon and I, like Job, could speak life into a dying situation because Proverbs 18:21 says, "Death and life are in the power of the tongue." We were compelled, then, to speak and breathe life to his bones.

We'd have to confront a potentially destructive disease and a ruthless adversary, but we've been given strong armor; the helmet of salvation, the breastplate of righteousness, and the mighty sword of the Spirit, the Word of God, which He esteems above His very name.

Jehovah instructed His people in Deuteronomy 11:18-21, to obey the Words of His commandments and instructions, to "lay up these words of Mine in your heart and in your soul, and bind them as a sign on your hand, and they shall be as frontlets between your eyes. And you shall teach them to your children, speaking of them when you sit in your house, and when you walk by the way, when you lie down and when you rise up. And you shall write them on the doorposts of your house, and on your gates, that your days and the days of your children may be multiplied..."

I believed the passage literally and searched for healing Scriptures, as well as those that applied to strengthening us and growing us up in His Word. I typed several of them in different script styles, printed them out, and posted them on many of our walls and doorposts so whenever I felt troubled or needed grace to help me in time of need, His

Word was ever before me to encourage me and fortify my trust in Him.

Those who are well have no need of a physician.
Matthew 9:12

Expert and compassionate care are as valuable as medicine. jmj

Chapter Fifteen

DOCTOR DAWSON

We sat in the new oncologist's examining room, anxious to meet with her. After his latest diagnosis, Euvon had made a decision to follow conventional therapy protocol, as suggested by his original doctor. I supported him in his decision, albeit with some reservations. We had stepped into a new world practically blindfolded, not knowing what to expect, completely at its mercy.

Yet, when she entered the room, Doctor Nancy Dawson greeted us with a smile she'd wear to embrace a friend, setting us at ease. I immediately liked her, confidant she would treat him with care.

She asked Euvon how he felt, to which he responded that he was experiencing some tingling radiating down his right leg, bone pain in his right hip, back pain and blurred vision, but otherwise, he felt great.

Wow.

Doctor Dawson explained that all of his tests confirmed stage IV metastatic prostate cancer which had spread to his bones and lymph nodes. The hormone therapy she prescribed for him, which would begin immediately, would be the best alternative, since chemotherapy and radiation would likely disturb his quality of life. The daily pill, Casodex, and the trimonthly Lupron shot would alleviate much of his discomfort, as well as block the testosterone hormone. He would also be given a monthly calcium shot, called Xgeva, as well as additional calcium and Vitamin D-3 supplements to help strengthen his bones. She expected this therapy to increase his appetite, which I appreciated because he had lost a dramatic amount of weight.

Once our meeting was over, we were sent to another department to receive his calcium and hormone shots. A nurse led us into an open room separated from the general public by a curtain. Euvon sat in his assigned lounge chair and engaged in small talk with her while she prepared the needle.

"Okay," I exhaled. "What's the needle for?" She didn't realize that not only did I hate them, I'd seen enough of them over the last few weeks. And I could tell when she instructed Euvon to take off his shirt that he was tired as well.

The needle contained Xgeva, she said, while inserting it into his arm, which made him stiffen straight as a board. She pulled it out just as quickly and he relaxed.

As soon as she left, a second nurse appeared with quite the professional smile, holding what looked like a ten-foot mass weapon of warfare. She told him to stand up, face the wall, and lean on the chair.

"Wait a minute," he hesitated. "Why do I have to lean over?"

"Because," she said, "This shot goes into your buttock."

"My buttock?" he whispered as loud as he could. "Do you mean, I have to pull down my pants?"

"Well, Mr. Jones, not all the way. But don't worry, we do this all the time."

He looked at me as I inched my way to the other side of the curtain. "Where are you going?"

"I can't watch," I admitted. "I love you, but you've got to be a big guy with this one."

But, I peeked in over the curtain to see anyway.

"You ready, Mr. Jones?" the smiling nurse asked rhetorically.

He pulled his pants down just below his spine, took a deep breath, faced the wall, and braced himself against the back of the chair.

The nurse jabbed him; he screeched, I jumped.

"Good job, Mr. Jones. You're done." With that, she left.

I returned and sat down. His eyes and lips were glued shut and he could barely buckle his belt.

"Did it hurt that bad?" I'd inadvertently asked the worse question I could think of.

"Oh, yeah," he answered, shaking his head. "And I have to do this every three months. Dag."

"I'm sorry." I was scared to hug him. So, I just touched his hand and waited with him until he felt comfortable enough to leave.

My heart bled for him because he had to go through this. I wanted to cry for him, too, because this would probably be one of the last times I would accompany him to these torture chambers. Nope, this was it. One of us had to hold down the fort and have dinner waiting for him when he got home.

Children are a heritage from the Lord, the fruit of the womb is a reward. Like arrows in the hand of a warrior, so are the children of one's youth.
Psalm 127:3-4

Children can be your greatest allies and defense when they are properly trained in the way they should go. We bless the Lord at all times for ours.
jmj

Chapter Sixteen

OUR CHILDREN

The first thing we did once the emotional smoke settled was contact our children, Tara, Cristina, T'hai, and Ryan. It was important for them to be informed about their father's health challenge and revisit their family history.

A few of their aunts and cousins had been diagnosed with breast cancer, while others, including myself, had reproductive cysts and tumors. Their paternal grandfather had been diagnosed with prostate cancer, and now their father. These illnesses have a propensity to be hereditary, and we wanted them to be better able to pray with wisdom and to know about available preventive measures, including getting regular checkups, participating in screenings, and making any necessary dietary changes.

My father-in-law had been raised in an era and in an environment where good healthcare for blacks was not easily attainable nor successful. And, my husband didn't remember getting regular checkups growing up. So, by the time he'd become a working adult and acquired quality health coverage, he rarely took advantage of it.

Euvon likened his body to what he believed most men could relate to - a new car. Of course, he knew what the Scriptures said about our bodies being God's temple, but most men, he said, drive their bodies similar to a car. They'll take their "car" anywhere it wants to go, even to places it shouldn't be, and they'll let it do things that shouldn't be done. They may put the wrong oil in it, if they add any at all, and burn the motor.

Men fail to realize that God only gives them one "car," and they don't get to trade it in during this life for another one. Their "car" doesn't really belong to them anyway. It belongs to the Lord, and one way He should be honored is by being good stewards over their bodies, which is their main driving force.

Euvon also believed that being used by God had a lot to do with stewardship, and taking care of his body should have been part of it. To ignore it was an arrogant way of living, something he felt he had done for much of his life.

So it was also critical to stress to our children the importance of having good health coverage and taking the necessary steps to maintain a healthy lifestyle.

When we finally talked with them, instead of bawling with sorrow as I did when I found out about Euvon's condition, they encouraged and assured us they would be available for whatever we needed. They laid hands on us and prayed warrior prayers, touching and agreeing that their father would be healed and I would be strengthened to do everything required of me as his helpmeet.

Jehovah Rapha is our Healer, they concluded, which settled it for them. That was it. Cut and dry. Hallelujah. Amen.

Ointment and perfume delight the heart,
and the sweetness of a man's friend gives
delight by hearty counsel.
Proverbs 27:9

As iron sharpens iron, so a man sharpens
the countenance of his friend.
Proverbs 27:17

Chapter Seventeen

FROM HERE TO ETERNITY

News spread fast about Euvon's diagnosis, and he soon received calls of shock and despair that someone as kind a person as he could have been diagnosed with such a devastating disease. There had to have been some mistake. But, no, we were facing a life changing battle, and they wanted to assist in any way they could. T'hai had already decided that she and her daughter, Tylind, would remain with us for a few weeks to help us adjust. So, we encouraged our closest family and friends to pray.

Before we knew it, cancer had become the topic of our conversation to almost anyone who would listen. Strangers were even allowed to peek into that part of our lives. We never knew if our story would encourage someone else, or whether we were talking to an angel in disguise sent by

God to impart some wisdom into us, to simply console us, or best of all, to heal him.

The more we talked about it, the more we realized how popular it was. One of my aunts used to quip, "You ain't in style if you don't have cancer." We used to laugh about it until now. Everyone we talked with had dealt with it in some way, either directly or indirectly. Once the "c" word was mentioned, it was as if the inner jar storing their trauma had suddenly cracked, oozing out the pain through their eyes and conversations, however brief.

There were recollections of how it was either kicked in the face and defeated, or how it became too powerful and destructive to wrestle loose its stronghold. We heard everything from, "He exercised two hours a day and ended up breaking a hip from brittle bones," or "Cancer pushed him down the stairs and broke his neck," or "She was on the brink of death, when suddenly she sat up, whole and healed!" Tales of tragedies and triumphs were exchanged in grocery lines, restaurants, and church.

Our church family became a great source of strength, and we reached out to every brother and sister in Christ we knew, from California to Maryland, from Florida to New York, from the sanctuary to the parking lot, to lock hearts and pray for Euvon's healing.

Then, the Holy Spirit stirred in us that His presence was always with us. He could be seen through the telephone calls and e-mails, the cards, the comfort and support from our circle of family and friends, and the care of his doctors. He brought us to a pleasant place where we appreciated how much Euvon was loved, enabling him to forge ahead.

Once, we stood at our back door admiring the lofty trees surrounding much of our home, trusting that as He cared for the birds fluttering between them, and the squirrels posing at the edge of their limbs, He would care for us, never leaving nor forsaking us.

Euvon, overwhelmed and unaccustomed to that kind of attention and care, cried.

The Trial of Stage IV Prostate Cancer

PART FOUR

The Trial Of Change

It's a mighty poor wind that
don't change.
Anonymous

Quality of life suffocates in the
stagnation of unhealthy nutrition,
inadequate exercise, and excessive
behavior.   jmj

Chapter Eighteen

YOU ARE WHAT YOU EAT

One thing I'd learned about cancer was that it thrives well in a sugary, acidic and inflammatory environment. It depletes the immune system of any power to ward off harmful invasions. So, we were going to have to develop a diet that would maximize his overall health, while minimizing any side effects of hormone therapy.

I sorted through a plethora of information specifically regarding prostate cancer-fighting diets that could fit our lifestyle and budget. Then, I listed every food Euvon loved and researched whether they had been beneficial or detrimental to him. I also searched for recipes online and in the many cookbooks I'd accumulated through the years that I could modify and incorporate to entice him away from our beloved Southern soul food diet.

Euvon's absolute favorite meal, a fat juicy rib-eye steak or filet mignon, baked potato slathered with butter, sour cream and chives, and toxic conventional salad was immediately out of the question; it was a recipe for disaster.

Several studies indicated that broiled or grilled steaks are exposed to chemical carcinogens when their juices mingle with an open flame. Conventional potatoes were also a culprit because as a root vegetable, they're grown in pesticide and insecticide-laden soil. And most of our salad vegetables, if not organic, produced a practically lethal side dish, not only because the lettuce, cucumbers, and carrots, to name a few, are drenched in pesticides and insecticides, but also because they were drizzled with a dressing full of high fructose corn syrup, sugar, and artificial ingredients.

Now I'm no serial killer, but I sulked over the possibility that every time I'd prepared that meal in the past, which was at least four or five times a month, I was shooting my husband right square in the prostate. The thought that with every bite, it was getting sicker and sicker, his immune system was shooting blanks, and the Spirit of God was shaking His head in pity, made me feel queazy.

Euvon's second favorite meal, peach or cherry cobbler, topped with ice cream, was the size of an entree. The desserts' main ingredient, sugar, and Euvon were cut buddies for life. It was in his coffee, in his sodas, and in the vending machines' processed cakes, pies, and chips he bought faithfully every day. I don't recall a time when we didn't store one of those items in our freezer or on our cabinet shelves. We always made a concerted effort to fill the void of missing sugar at first glance.

Our frequent dinners of fried chicken, potato salad, and pork-seasoned greens was another pernicious meal we enjoyed. I couldn't believe how damaging our food choices had been to our bodies.

Euvon also loved seafood but, by golly, our personal selections were as substandard as the fish themselves. We often dined on what we considered the elite, chilean sea bass, ahi tuna, shark, and swordfish. But, their levels of mercury matched their exorbitant prices, which only added to our contamination. We also ate the cheap salmon injected with some added mysterious color. Since we were Marylanders, the ever acidic steamed, broiled, or fried shellfish, including our beloved blue crabs, lobsters, mussels, shrimp, and oysters were also an absolute no-brainer.

Once I became aware that some of our most loved foods were actually our most hated enemies, not only because of how they were prepared, but also because of the frequency in which we indulged, I had to make a decision.

Those frequent favorites, as well as fried pork chops or beef liver smothered in onions, garlic, green onions and gravy, with mashed potatoes and butter, and sweet peas. Gone.

Broiled lobster, dipped in lemon-butter, baked potato loaded with butter and sour cream, and salad filled with pesticides, insecticides, and high fructose corn syrup. Gone.

Deep fried lake trout, deep fried french fries, high fructose corn syrup cole slaw. Gone.

Deep fried shrimp, chicken, and scallop tempura. Gone.

Decadent homemade cakes, pies, cookies. Gone.

Homemade ice-cream, with extra eggs and sugar. Gone.

Every food that seduced the palate. Gone.

No, I had to create a way to wean us into a more nutritious diet without much scrutiny and, if he did notice, without a dog fight. An almost impossible task lay ahead, but I had to embrace it. Yet, regardless of what I prepared or how I prepared it at this fourth stage of the game of advanced prostate cancer, without the hand of God stirring the pot, it wouldn't matter. With Him, though, I thought we'd make a great team.

Chapter Nineteen

"I WANT REAL FOOD"

One day, I suggested we try organic foods. I'd read many times over that it was the best option for healthy eating, and I wanted to incorporate it into our lives. Although it was more expensive than conventional foods, it was much cheaper than doctors' bills.

I had experimented with it during my own health challenges a few years before, and I could feel a difference in my stamina. While Euvon thought the idea was "cute," he preferred sticking with what he knew. Taste and pizzaz. Suggesting the whole organic thing in the past, like it was a pie-in-the-sky way to health was a hard thing to sell to him because he'd never been sick.

Now, though, he was still struggling with some physical discomfort, as well as with his appetite and at a point where he no longer enjoyed eating the foods he loved. So I thought this would be a good time to wean him into something different.

"Besides," I reasoned, "we've been eating a lot of toxins, and we've spent a ton of money trashing ourselves with junk. Our bodies have now spoken, and we've become human landfills. I honestly believe if we eat healthier, you'll have the strength you need during your therapy. And I believe the Lord would approve of it."

The moment I spoke God's Name, Euvon became more agreeable.

So I started with chicken noodle soup. It had often been the stuff that soothed the savage stomach in our home, especially the one not wanting the trouble of digesting anything anyway. Whenever a cold or flu challenged Euvon's appetite, I'd fix him a big pot of homemade chicken noodle soup. It made him feel better, and he'd quickly improve. So, that was it.

Substituting conventional ingredients with organic ones, I prepared the soup as I usually did - slicing, chopping, sautéing, simmering - and presented my labor of love to him on a tray while he rested and watched television.

Euvon studied the soup, sniffed it, scooped a bit onto his spoon, blew, and sipped. Then he gave me a look that made me think I had served him raw rats. He got up, marched to the kitchen, and grabbed the box of salt and the jar of sugar. I snatched the jar from him, which he replaced with a bottle of sugar and junk filled Worcestershire sauce. No sooner had I removed the salt from the other hand, he had picked up the jar of sugar again.

"No sugar," I demanded, taking it from him again.

Before I knew it, he banged his fist on the counter and burst into tears, crying like a newborn baby.

"What am I supposed to do? I can't eat that stuff! I'm doing the best I can!"

Startled, all I could answer was, "But you haven't eaten yet."

"Well, I don't want to eat that," he wailed louder and slumped over the counter. "It doesn't even taste like food!"

Oh, really? Well, I set the salt, Worcestershire sauce, and sugar on the counter in front of him and stomped out of the kitchen.

"Fine. Hurt yourself."

I slammed our bedroom door and sat on the bed. Resentful and humiliated, I started tearing up myself. How dare he not even pretend to like the soup I toiled over just for him. How dare he treat me like I was worse than cancer itself.

I felt as though I'd failed him over something as simple as a stupid bowl of chicken noodle soup. And when I failed him, I failed. I cried and sulked, promising myself that would be the last bowl of soup he would taste from that kitchen. As a matter of fact, why don't we just forget this whole organic stuff? Why don't we just toxin it up? Pardon me for only trying to help. Forget it. I don't care what we do….Fast foods and…….

Through the muck and mire of my thoughts, though, through the thin bedroom walls, I could still hear him crying. And for the first time, I sensed a man who sounded tired and fearful.

"Father," I asked, "what's happened over a simple bowl of chicken noodle soup?" I wanted to go to Euvon, but I still held on to a fraction of annoyance. So I just listened until every wail brushed away the fraction, erasing everything but sorrow. It dawned on me, then, that this wasn't really about the soup - no, it was much bigger. The life we'd become accustomed to for most of our marriage was over. If we had not apprehended it before, we sure were now hit with the reality and conundrum of a devastating diagnosis, a rerouted future, and distorted plans. The walls of our strength had finally breached, and a flood of helpless and fearful tears gushed out of us.

All those terrifying emotions finally gave way to fatigue. So, I got up, opened the door, and walked down the hall to him. As I tried to relax beside him, he whined, "I'm sorry, I'm sorry."

Our world had come to a halt that night until the cries subsided, and an air of quiet peace breezed through our tired souls. All we could do, then, was rest our heads against each other.

Then, I embraced him and held on to him. He leaned his head on my shoulder, and while he softly groaned on the outside, I screamed and moaned on the inside.

*So, whether you eat or drink, or
whatever you do, do it all for the glory
of God.*
1 Corinthians 10:31

Chapter Twenty

NUTRITION

Well, moaning and groaning about it wasn't going to change anything. We still had to kiss our old way of living good-bye and, without being too dogmatic, transition into a healthier lifestyle. I was a novice who was going to have to rely on books and social media to educate me because for us, time was a precious commodity, and I didn't think I had enough of it to take long, drawn-out classes, workshops, or seminars.

So, I prayed for the Holy Spirit to stir my mind and give me wisdom. While my husband girded his loins and appetite and pushed ahead to continue providing for us, I delved into the world of organic and natural foods, compiling as much information as I could from the countless internet conversations and controversies regarding organic versus conventional, raw versus cooked, and meat versus vegetarian versus vegan eating.

And, there was an equal amount of reports and books about the thousand and one diets that needed to be incorporated, including the Mediterranean diet, the Japanese diet, the low-fat, high fiber diet, the raw diet, the diabetic diet, and on and on and on. The majority concluded that meat, pasta, and breads belonged at the bottom of the food chain, while seafood, fruits, and vegetables were the creme de la creme.

What concerned me, though, were the caveats about the many important fruits, vegetables, nuts, and seeds we've eaten most of our lives being contaminated with dangerously generous amounts of pesticides and insecticides that weaken our immune systems, and promote illness and disease. Most of these fruit and nut trees, as well as many garden vegetables, were thought to live in toxic conditions, with their growers being accused of having little regard for their effect on our wellbeing. Then, they're processed and stored in toxic metal cans, labeled with a host of unpronounceable, artificial ingredients that scream at us, and shipped off to supermarkets, including some organic ones, for us consumers to snap up and ingest.

Further, our foods, especially meats, are supposedly wrapped in poisonous plastics like cling wrap and styrofoam. These two kinds, classified as #6, along with #3 and #7 plastics, are considered the most toxic because they contain certain human carcinogenic chemicals that could leach into foods and, therefore, into our bodies. And they were practically everywhere in my freezer and cabinets. Plastics labeled #1, #2, #4, and #5, while deemed safer, still weren't completely exonerated.

No wonder, then, that within years for some, and in no time at all for others, obesity, illness, disease, and other physical and mental disorders become the norm, with the majority of society feeding on some kind of medication.

So, after weighing all the pros and cons, and erring on the side of caution, I made some executive decisions about what would be best for us and began a household overhaul.

I threw out almost every toxic plastic container in my kitchen, including the ones with no numbered labels just to be sure. I opted for glass storage containers and was pleasantly surprised to see that foods, especially organic produce, which tended to deteriorate before I could transport it from the store to the refrigerator, preserved better and longer in them.

Any canned, frozen, or packaged food consisting of an ingredient I couldn't pronounce, or containing any form of sugar, especially high fructose corn syrup and artificial sweeteners were tossed. We replaced white flour, sugar, and pasta with organic versions and added other grains, like buckwheat, spelt, quinoa, and millet. Organic olive oil, which I call Abba's oil, since it is highly regarded in the Bible, became our main oil for sautéing and making salad dressings. We also used homemade organic clarified butter, or ghee, and coconut, sesame, and avocado oils. Vegetable oil and margarine were out.

We replaced sodas with filtered, alkaline water, and herbal teas, experimenting with different flavors. Euvon's favorites and most nourishing were green, white, rooibus, hibiscus, milk thistle, and peppermint teas. We opted to continue drinking coffee, but brewed it with organic beans I would grind almost daily.

Vitamins and supplements, such as Vitamins C and D-3, Co-Q 10, Calcium Citrate, along with Milk Thistle, Astragalus, Maitake Mushroom, Reishi Mushroom, and Immune Defense tinctures also became a part of our regimen.

Since Euvon's health and immune system had already been severely compromised and needed a major boost, I took inventory of the best organic foods that were most beneficial for him, as well as the least contaminated conventional foods still considered healthy.

During the winter, we stocked up on frozen berries and red grapefruit which reportedly contained healthy antioxidants and the least amount of sugar.

Cruciferous vegetables, including red and green cabbage, napa and savoy cabbage, bok choy, brussel sprouts, kale, collards, arugula, radishes, horseradish, daikon radishes, broccoli, cauliflower, and watercress, as well as yams, more than other potatoes, were included in our diet because they contained a greater level of nutrients.

Once spring and summer arrived, we frequented organic supermarkets and local farmers' markets in search of fresh, colorful organic produce. We even bought and prepared some we'd never heard of but were excited to try, like meyer lemons, garlic scape, kohlrabi, and purple sweet potatoes. We also splurged on fresh organic berries, cherries, and grapes. Cherries were as important as they were delicious because I'd read they contain a group of compounds called anthocynins, which may encourage tumor cells to kill themselves without hurting the healthy cells. So, along with the fresh cherries, we bought tart cherry juice concentrate and added two tablespoons to water, juice, or our favorite smoothies almost daily.

Grapes were also important because their skins contain resveratrol, which is believed to be a potent antioxidant. Grapes are also used to make red wine, which the Apostle

Paul advised his protege, Timothy, in First Timothy 5:23, to drink in small amounts, saying, "No longer drink only water, but use a little wine for your stomach's sake and your frequent illnesses," and we would sometimes end our day with a glass or two ourselves.

Euvon and I included many of the acceptable conventional fruits, such as melons, mangos, kiwi, and bananas, since their outer layers protected them from those nasty toxins. We often froze most of our fruits and used them for smoothies or as toppings for pancakes or waffles, yogurt, and cereal.

Meat eating was an issue warranting Abba's perspective, because depending on what circle you were in, it was either deadly and the main cause of sickness, or it was nutritious in small amounts. Some swore God never intended for us to eat meat or wear clothes or shoes made with animal skins. Others believed we were given the grace to eat whatever we want, as long as we said Grace.

So I went to the Bible for advice and read in Genesis 1:29-30, that after God made man and the other living creatures, their diets consisted of plants and fruits alone. He said to man, "I have given you every herb that yields seed which is on the face of all the earth, and every tree whose fruit yields seed; to you it shall be for food. Also, to every beast of the earth, to every bird of the air, and to everything that creeps on the earth, in which there is life, I have given every green herb for food."

But then, according to Genesis 3, Adam and Eve committed the infamous sin, eating from the tree of the knowledge of good and evil; so, God initiated the first sacrifice of an animal to atone for their sin and to clothe them with its skin.

By Genesis 9:3, the whole world had become so decrepit and wicked, the Lord caused a great flood to rid the earth of degradation, saving only the righteous Noah, his family, and two of every kind of creature upon the earth so they could reproduce and multiply. Then, He instructed Noah saying, "Every moving thing that lives shall be food for you. I have given you all things, even as the green herbs."

In Exodus 16, God Himself supernaturally fed His people manna and quail. Then in Leviticus 11, He specified to Moses other meats He approved of for His people to eat. The slaughter of those animals, though, were to be performed as painless and humane as possible, contrary to what's being done today.

God gave us dominion over animals, and while I believe they can be used for food and clothing, they are also to be treated with respect.

Many corporations who transfer their conventional meats from their poisonous barns and gestation crates to our mouths today treat their animals in a disgraceful manner. Some livestock are injected with arsenic and other poisons to prevent disease and promote growth. Others are crammed in filthy gestation crates, making it impossible for them to do anything except wait to be artificially impregnated repeatedly for most of their lives and push out their young for the owners to poison up and feed to the consumer.

This troubling information forced Euvon and me to purchase ninety-five percent organic meat and five percent grass-fed. Since it fell to the bottom of the food chain, we simply ate less of it and doubled up on fruits, vegetables, good carbs, and seafood.

I flavored bland foods with different kinds of sea salt, including sea salt flakes, Himalayan pink salt, grey salt, and fleur de sel, and added an abundance of herbs and spices, including basil, thyme, cilantro, cinnamon, cumin, and tumeric, which also contain nutritional properties.

Our palates gradually began to appreciate organic textures and tastes, making quite an impression on us, and leaving us less sluggish and bloated after meals. Euvon's endurance increased, while I inadvertently shed a few unwanted pounds.

Chapter Twenty-one

SUSTAINABLE LIVING

I got so excited about the difference our new diet had made on Euvon and me, I rolled up my sleeves and dug deeper to explore beyond the kitchen and figure out other ways to live healthier.

I knew that our skin is our largest organ, and the products we use for daily hygiene alone seep into our pores and lymph nodes, circulating any poisonous chemical throughout our bodies. Euvon's bones and lymph nodes were already under attack, and I wanted to know what his body had been exposed to from the inside out.

So, I walked through every room and examined almost everything that included questionable ingredients and materials, from skin and hair care products, to medicines and bandages, from bedding to shower curtains, from carpets to cleaning products.

It was an overwhelming endeavor because I could see that almost everything we owned was stored in toxic plastic, or contained at least one potentially harmful ingredient. Some of our clothes even smelled like they had been made with chemicals, especially many of those labeled, "made in China." And, something as unnoticeable as our plastic shower curtains and liners, were found to be toxic because of some carcinogenic chemical called PVC. I threw away some of our blended clothes in favor of cotton and linen, and bought fabric shower curtains and liners.

But even then, completely eradicating toxins from our home meant blowing it up and rebuilding something more organic and eco-friendly.

While I crave a sterile and lofty existence along some rolling hill with clean, fresh air, lush fruit and nut trees, and beautiful herb and vegetable gardens, I could only settle for what was possible now to minimize this current deadly stalking. I had enough information stored away about eco-friendly and sustainable living to try to make as many somewhat educated decisions as possible to improve our environment as I had regarding our nutrition.

The blessing in my life was that I had always been an artsy craftsy kind of person. I remember playing in the dirt as a young toddler, making mud pies and cakes, so much so that I was labeled "the little dirt diaper." As I got older, my sister called me Holly Hobbit because I loved baking from scratch, designing my own clothes, and creating unique ceramic decor for our home.

So I believed I could translate that kind of creativity into making some of our own personal and household products. Once again, I relied on the internet for guidance, which helped me produce a collection of what I considered healthy body and hair recipes.

I also learned that vodka, white vinegar, and tea tree oil served as dependable non-toxic replacements for cleaning products full of poisonous fumes, as well as antiseptic and anti-fungal relief for simple cuts and insect bites. Sometimes I would combine vodka with equal parts of water and about twenty drops of lemon, orange, lavender, or peppermint oil to use as an air or linen freshener.

Whatever I didn't have the nerve to make, such as body soap, shampoo, fabric and dish detergent, I bought with as many natural ingredients as possible.

While I couldn't prove that anything I'd done was going to improve my husband's quality of life, I rested in those small lifestyle changes because even if it didn't, it certainly would not have lessened that quality.

I knew there would be times when we would relax and cheat, but such is life. For the most part, though, I believed we could discipline ourselves to this new way of life, work out our faith and fight a good fight.

Chapter Twenty-two

CHOICES

Once Euvon settled into his hormone therapy routine, I asked him how he'd felt about our diet change and the progress he'd made so far.

He made it clear that in the beginning, he felt like I was some evil god who had dragged him around hell by his feet. It didn't matter that he had no appetite; he still loved the foods he'd eaten most of his adult life and looked forward to enjoying them again.

But since it wasn't going to happen with me in the kitchen, he had to get used to it. Initially, he said, some organic foods had interesting textures and tastes, but for the most part, eating was rather bland and unlikable. However, as much as he disliked this new lot in life, he had an equal fear of the foods he loved which could have been detrimental for him to eat. And it would have been presumptuous to be so driven by his passion that he would engage in a sugary risk just to satisfy his compulsion.

Euvon's most important desire was to live, but he also knew that wanting to live, yet doing it his way, didn't match. He couldn't tell God he was going to do something, although he knew what he was doing could kill him; and then, if he were dying, tell Him He'd let him down because he wanted to live.

God's grace has given us the opportunity in the midst of our diagnoses to change. We've also been given choices, which have everything to do with what we want. Before Euvon knew of his condition, he had been hard bent on doing what he wanted when he wanted to because it worked, and there was no need for change.

But after being smacked in the face with the realization of his life's fragility and his condition's severity, he understood that if he wanted to live, he would have to make some life changes, and diet was one of them.

He'd now come to enjoy it, though, because it allowed him to be more proactive in his quality of life. He also believed if he stayed the course and did what he needed to do - eating right, exercising, taking hot showers to soothe his achy bones, and avoiding toxic exposure whenever possible, by the Lord's goodness and mercy, he would be healed.

So I felt somewhat confidant my work was paying off, which encouraged me to continue searching for interesting recipes and solutions to help us thrive well in a rather challenging and toxic world.

The Trial of Stage IV Prostate Cancer

PART FIVE

THE CLINICAL TRIAL

OF

IMMUNOTHERAPY

Hope deferred makes the heart sick.
Proverbs 13:12

Chapter Twenty-three

WHAT'S NEXT?

By early spring, the Casodex pill, and the Xgeva and Lupron shots had alleviated Euvon's pain, returned his appetite to normal, and decreased that venomous psa level from 398 to 0.1, which rendered it undetectable. We were so elated, we imagined ourselves floating above cloud nine and touching a rainbow. We breathed a hallelujah sigh of relief and celebrated with a nice dinner at a quaint little organic restaurant in South Baltimore.

Everything seemed to be falling into place. The medicines were working, and our modified lifestyle appeared effective. Except for hot flashes and occasional mild groin pain, he showed no sign of sickness.

But it was all short-lived and written in the wind sooner than we expected. During one of his exams a few short weeks later, it was discovered that his psa level had become detectable again, and his doctor wanted to re-exam him in two weeks. But, by then, it had risen once more. A couple of weeks later, when it had risen yet again, the doctor concluded that the Casodex was no longer effective. Euvon seemed to take the news in stride, unalarmed because his psa level had been elevated before, and he didn't even know he had cancer. It didn't matter if it was one, fifty, or three hundred, he had felt no signs of the disease. It took his psa level to reach 398 for it to manifest itself. And when he started hormone therapy, his level dropped to an undetectable level.

He was no longer in the kind of pain that brought him to the doctor in the first place. He was still strong and active, and he'd spent much time in prayer. So he assumed his psa level had increased because of what the cancer was doing in his body. He had not had a bone scan lately; so, no one but the Lord knew how it was behaving.

"God is in control, knowing what to do," he insisted, "So, what's next?"

I, on the other hand, felt a death grip and needed to consult with the Lord. For some reason, I felt this latest setback had been my fault. What could I have possibly done wrong? Was it too much of this, not enough of that? Had I not been dedicated enough to his wellness? Had I researched in all the wrong places without consulting the experts? The few whose advice I had sought in the past, had little else to offer, except, "Just let him eat whatever he wants," or, "Let him do whatever he wants." What they were really saying was, "Look, he's dying; so, whatever."

So, what happened? Had we not prayed enough? Had the adversary kicked our faith down the stairs without our knowing, because we weren't paying enough attention to it anyway? Had I really been reading healing Scriptures through jaundiced lenses, memorizing them, without truly meditating on them? Were my occasional tears those of joy or resolve? Was my faith hopeful or jaded, which nullified faith altogether?

I waited for answers. I heard none. It took some time, but I finally conceded that Abba was not always going to talk me through this trial. He was going to walk me through it, and He was going to walk Euvon through it. We would just have to feel our way to find His steady hand, grasp it, and trust the path He was leading us.

But at that moment, listening to the doctor, all I could see was death and defeat trying to crash our health party, and me throwing everything organic out the window.

Let the probing, "What?" dispel the frightening, "Why?"

jmj

Chapter Twenty-four

ASYMPTOMATIC METASTATIC CASTRATE REFRACTORY

See, Euvon had now entered the ASYMPTOMATIC METASTATIC CASTRATE REFRACTORY phase of stage IV prostate cancer. In a nutshell, he had become resistant to his existing hormone therapy, and the Casodex had to be removed from his treatment. Thankfully, chemotherapy and radiation still weren't considered. But, what was next?

Doctor Dawson suggested that since he was asymptomatic, with no side effects other than hot flashes and a hearty appetite, he could probably qualify for some clinical trial in which his own immune system would be used to combat the disease. The only other catch was that his psa level would have to be within the range of between four and nineteen. Sometimes, she advised, once the Casodex is removed from therapy, the psa level could fall below four and become normal again, in which case, he would not qualify for, nor need to undergo the trial.

In the meantime, we received two thick packets of complicated information about the clinical trial to digest and discuss with our children. We had welcomed every opportunity to involve them because it wasn't something Euvon and I wanted to face alone. Our entire family was attacking this enemy, and we wanted as much of their involvement as possible. Besides, perhaps, one of us could decipher one portion of the contents, while another could comprehend a different aspect. If all else failed, Euvon had a kind, caring, and respected oncologist, who delivered as much truth as she felt we could handle at any given moment.

We tried to make sense of the gist of this trial. It involved a six-week immunotherapy program, in which on one day, for three to four hours, Euvon would undergo a process called leukapheresis, given at a blood center, where some of his blood would be extracted from his body and passed through a machine. The machine would then collect a small amount of his healthy immune cells, platelets, and red blood cells, and return the remaining cells and blood to his body. Those cells would then be shipped to an FDA-approved manufacturing facility where, over the course of two to three days, it would be processed with a solution of nutrients, becoming his own unique dose of Provenge. Euvon would then report to the hospital three days later, where it would be infused back into his system with the hope that it would quicken his immune system enough to fight the cancer. Timing was crucial in order to keep the cells active while waiting for the infusion process.

Euvon would then rest a week. The second series would be repeated the following week, followed by a week of rest. The final phase would begin and end the following week, with an additional week of rest, totaling six weeks.

Euvon loved the idea that cells could be collected from his body and used to cause his body to buffet his own body. He reasoned that once he got to know cancer, he realized its cells, once healthy, had gone haywire, beating up on the remaining good ones. So some of the good cells would be rescued and fed special nutrients. Then, they would be infused back into his body ready to wage war against the bad cells - the good guys versus the bad guys.

While the treatment sounded great, I was more skeptical of the side effects. At the same time, he had, so far, been blessed with minimal issues. He diligently continued his business with an upbeat attitude, believing that if God be for him, nothing nor no one could stand against him. So our children and I determined to stand with him in faith.

By his next hospital visit, and before we could decide whether he would be involved with the clinical trial, Euvon's oncologist notified him that his psa level had fallen below four; therefore, he wouldn't qualify to participate in the clinical trial. Apparently, as his body cleared itself of the pill, his level returned to almost normal, as predicted. He was only required to endure the calcium and Lupron shots. Praise God!

The Trial of Stage IV Prostate Cancer

A longing fulfilled is a tree of life.
Proverbs 13:12

Chapter Twenty-five

LIFE

Euvon and I had dodged a bullet and took advantage of this reprieve. We'd also considered life from another perspective, which meant spending more time with each other while we were still somewhat healthy. So, he decreased his business hours and rested more so we could explore a little more of our world together.

I suggested we create a bucket list of small adventures we'd like to do that we've never done before. Nothing fancy or longwinded, since Euvon still had frequent appointments with his oncologist and needed to be close to home for the most part. So, just something the two of us could enjoy together or with others.

Well, he rebuked that in Jesus' Name. He had no intention on creating a bucket list of any kind, nor had he planned to kick the bucket any time soon. He preferred experiencing L.I.F.E, Living in Full Expectation, and creating latter-year memories.

Within a month, we were gifted with the opportunity to attend a Metropolitan Opera performance with our daughter, Cristina. Not just any performance, but the performance of a lifetime. We were about to witness our seven-year-old granddaughter, Ryen, grace the stage for a few precious moments with some of the greatest operatic voices in the world, one of whom happened to be one of our lifelong friends.

I had planned, off and on, for many years to attend one of her performances, but as the Lord would have it, this would be the first time Euvon and I would see our friend, together with our granddaughter, perform. Amidst the grandeur of the production, I sat in awe of Abba's precision, never opening the door for us to enter the Met's grand theater until that very moment. We would attend again, a few months later when, for the first time, Ryen's sister, Jordan, would also perform on that great stage.

We ended up traveling to New York more than we'd ever done in our lifetime to see them, along with our third granddaughter, Tylind, perform in several musical and theater productions with The Harlem School of the Arts.

Then, there was the trip to Virginia, where our oldest granddaughter, Symone, graduated from a historically black college with a degree in Vocal Performance and Education. She also became a member of the Virginia Opera Company, and we were blessed to see a few of her productions.

One Thanksgiving, we prepared and enjoyed an exclusive organic dinner with our children and grandchildren, which competed heavily with our conventional holiday meals. Then, we hosted a New Year's Eve party for the first time in our marriage. We also, at times, prepared organic meals and delivered them to a few family and friends who weren't feeling well.

One day, hubby and I decided to drive to a local home furnishing store we often enjoyed meandering through, to buy a few odds and ends. What started out as a small shopping spree ended up becoming an investment in kitchen cabinetry.

We'd been wanting to give our kitchen a makeover for years, anyway, because it had been occupied more than any other room. But, it was old, with dark, worn cabinets that looked tired of being opened and slammed shut for the past twenty years. The white countertops were stained and scratched beyond repair. We needed more space and desired more beauty but never found the time nor the inclination to prioritize home improvement over vacations and living a limited carefree lifestyle.

Euvon also refused to allow anyone to renovate his home when he could do it himself. He took home-improvement seriously and nothing short of death would deter him from his "do-it-myself" adventures.

Almost ten years ago, he had practically severed his wrist while transporting thin layers of sheet metal to a job site. His nerves and bones required surgical repair, and he endured over a year of grueling physical therapy. Yet, he believed there was no better way to speed his healing and strengthen his wrist than to literally single-handedly build an extension to our deck.

I was of little help then, because I thought he'd lost his mind. But, he worked diligently at balancing each wooden board on one shoulder while he hammered nails with unsteady fingers and wobbly wrists. Instead of complaining, he whistled while he worked, and today, our addition is as sturdy as it was the day he hammered the last nail to its completion.

Now, we thought this would be another therapeutic time to remodel our kitchen. So, Euvon transformed into a one-man construction company who would upgrade our prehistoric looking room into something brighter, more modern and spacious, while I remained the one-woman chef, sautéing, steaming, and baking away. We rolled up our sleeves and let the work begin.

For the next few months, Euvon would come home from work and dive right into measuring, cutting, and hammering. Sometimes, we'd step back and examine the progress; then detour, tear down, level and plum, repair, sand, scrape, clean, shop, sometimes with "Heaven's, that's the wrong size," return shop, "Oops, it cracked," more purchases, level and plumb, hammer and nails, and paint.

Then, one day, we finally stood in the midst of our "new" kitchen, admiring the fruit of our labor, appreciating its beauty. It had been a labor of love, and our relationship had become more enriched. Other than our marriage, it had been the longest project we'd ever undertaken involving just the two of us, and we were happy we'd once again experienced "LIFE."

Together, we'd witnessed the day-by-day transformation of our little kitchen into a place we were especially proud of. There had been errors along the way but, hey, it was our kitchen, and our aesthetic view included those errors, of which we were also proud.

Our makeover reminded me of what I must look like from time to time from Abba's perspective - an old, outdated room with worn, unclean hands, and stained, impure thoughts. But, instead of trashing me in favor of a new model, He cuts and prunes, tears down and builds up, levels and plumbs, renews and restores, encouraging me to eat from the Bread of Life and meditate on His Word.

This particular LIFE venture distracted us from bouts of anxiety and uncertainty for a while and prepared us for the next phase of our lives that hit us from left field sooner than we expected.

Chapter Twenty-six

CLINICAL TRIAL

We thought it would have been nice to have received a little hint from Heaven that our happiness was about to change again, but God is almighty, and He does as He pleases. And a simple call was all it took.

Euvon's psa count had climbed again, another bone scan was needed, and we were faced with the immunotherapy we thought was behind us.

Euvon had been weaving his past hospital visits and injections in with his work days; so, I rarely went with him. And such was the case when he went to take the bone scan. The results, he said, indicated that there was no significant change in the locations nor the intensity of the cancer. It had not diminished but, praise God, it had not spread. His doctor encouraged him to simply continue his regular routine. He would, though, have to begin immunotherapy as soon as the holiday season ended. Since his birthday was January 5th, he insisted on waiting until after then, to which his doctor reluctantly agreed.

Christmas, New Year's, and his birthday three-stepped in and out like a waltz, and now it was time to brace ourselves for the immunotherapy. A few days before the initial treatment, Dendreon, the company that processed the blood cells, was thoughtful enough to ship Euvon a box of goodies, including a backpack containing a knit cap, a water bottle, antibacterial hand soap, lotion, lip balm, ear plugs, an eye mask, a book of puzzles, and a calendar book. We felt like he belonged to a special group of men who would receive special treatment, and we were touched by these small gifts.

Dendreon also called the day before to remind us of our responsibility to be prompt, and to bring all the proper identification. We could not be a minute late for any of the sessions.

The cell collection staff greeted us warmly and made us feel comfortable. Euvon's ID was checked at almost every entrance. Once we arrived at the treatment room, I sat directly across from my husband, who settled in a comfortable "easy" chair. I also faced a massive machine I assumed would extract his cells. The technician again checked his ID with the label that would be attached to his cell package for travel.

Euvon relaxed while the technician prepped his arms. As she connected the lumens to the machine, she explained that a needle would be inserted in or near the inner elbow of each arm. Blood would be drawn from one arm into the machine, which would collect a small amount of immune cells, platelets, and red blood cells. The remaining blood would be returned to his body through the needle in the other arm.

Well, no sooner than the first attempt was made to insert the needle into Euvon's left arm did all hell break loose. There were no veins large enough for the needle, and all he could do was grimace in pain each time she attempted to slide it into his arm. And no wonder. It was twice the size and width of the one used to draw his blood every month for tests.

When all of her attempts failed, she called upon a young colleague who she felt would have better success. Well, he may have been young, strong, and black, but he was no match against the massive needle and those thin veins that refused to cooperate. And as much as he was determined to shove that weapon into Euvon's vein, it just wasn't going to happen.

So they rested that arm and lodged an attack on the other one. Regardless of Euvon's growing discomfort and anxiety from all the poking and sticking, the technician tried all the tricks she'd used on the left arm with the right one. Well, Lordy, at one point, every prick left him stiff and groaning.

Finally, apparently as tired and frustrated as he, she jammed the needle into his arm. Blood splattered everywhere. He yelled, she hopped two steps backwards, and I jumped out of my seat.

The technician immediately teared up and apologized, believing it was her fault his arms were black and blue for naught. She finally concluded there would be no treatment that day because his veins were just too weak to handle a needle.

Euvon consoled and encouraged her, quickly tossing the ordeal behind him. He assured her it wasn't her fault at all. There was a time when his muscles were firm and rich with protruding veins. But, he was older now and had not exercised as much as he used to. Anyway, he assumed the Lord must not have wanted him to have the immunotherapy that day and gave him his daily dose of grace.

He thanked her for doing the best job she could with what she had to work with, and we bolted out the door, scared yet relieved.

But what now?! His veins were weak and options, few.

Within hours, Dr. Dawson was on the phone with Euvon, concluding that the clinical trial must proceed; however, since his veins were too weak, a Central Venus catheter would have to be inserted into his chest, which would allow him to receive his treatment. And no, he couldn't stop by her office on the way to work and get it done. It would require anesthesia and recovery.

This entire procedure meant that I would have to go with him. I was satisfied though because, on one hand, I needed to be with him to see for myself that a catheter placed in his chest was routine, nothing serious. On the other hand, it was so hard to see my husband at the complete mercy of strangers. But since he had to face the music, I figured I could, too.

Back at the hospital the following week, Euvon tried to divert his focus away from the uncomfortable needle pricks in his arm for the IV by asking questions. How long was the surgery going to last? What exactly were they going to do? When would he be able to eat, since he had not eaten anything after an early dinner the evening before? Could he return to work the next day? Blah, blah, blah.

His questions were answered quite nonchalantly, until they came to the part about what specifically needed to be done. His surgeon explained that the catheter would be inserted through Euvon's jugular vein and, excuse me? Y'all gonna mess with my husband's jugular?! Well, get the fools outta here! What happened to the simple forty-five minute stick-it-in-his-chest procedure?

No, the surgeon continued, it would take approximately three hours to insert the tube down his jugular vein and out through an opening in his chest. In the end, though, he would be able to receive the immunotherapy treatments without the nuisance of iffy pokings and prickings. Before, had he missed one treatment because a good vein could not be found, he would have had to begin again from square one. So, this was the best way to ensure his treatments would flow smoothly. We were assured he would be fine during the procedure and could leave as soon as he was awake and steady on his feet.

As he was being wheeled out of the room, I was offered an opportunity to relax and dine in a nearby cafe on the Georgetown University campus that served hospital staff, visitors, and university students and faculty. So, I blew him a kiss and ventured through the maze of hallways, passing by staff, visitors, and patients, wondering what some of them may have encountered that day.

Had that doctor just performed a successful operation? Was that woman confined to a wheelchair because of an accident or some debilitating illness? Or, bless the Lord, was that a proud daddy who had come to gather mommy and new baby for their journey home? Had this man, passing solemnly by, stood at the side of his loved one, waiting patiently for eyes to open, slipping away for a brief reprieve?

Although it was less than a five-minute walk, I felt as if I had traveled a hundred miles to another hemisphere, entering a cafe that, although buzzing with hungry and ambitious university students, left me suddenly feeling isolated and overwhelmed, searching for answers.

I really wanted to retrace my steps back to the operating room and just sit near Euvon to make sure they were taking care of him.

Instead, I purchased a light salad and pulled out the laptop I'd decided to bring at the last minute, deciding to catch up on being depressed about something else other than Euvon's operation. There were millions of people who had it worse than we, and someone was talking or writing about it on the Internet.

After I strayed, I repented.... I was ashamed and humiliated...
Jeremiah 31:19

What a wretched man I am! Who will rescue me from this body of death?...Therefore there is now no condemnation for those who are in Christ Jesus!
Romans 7:24; 8:1

Chapter Twenty-seven

REFLECTION

But then, I caught myself. I didn't want to read about someone else's sorrows just to appease my own. My soul longed after God now.

A few years after we'd joined our church's praise and worship team, one of our assistant pastors relocated to Northern Virginia to pastor an extension of our California church. Since it was close to our Maryland hometown, we followed and became involved in his music ministry.

Some of my family members, with whom I was eager to reunite, were unaccustomed to this new Christian and her "she-thinks-she's-perfect" lifestyle change, and we regularly clashed to a feverish pitch. I found myself frequently trying to prove to them that I wasn't as perfect as their accusations, and before I knew it, I had wearied myself out of church altogether, loosening my hold on the Lord and latching on to much of my "before Christ" days. I had backslidden faster than a scooter racing unmanned downhill, and the seams of my life had ripped apart like poorly sewn fabric, baring a disjointed relationship with everyone, including the Lord.

Then, increased family turbulence, including the deaths of my mother and sister, brought me to one of the lowest points of my life. One night, drenched in tears and alcohol, I vaguely remembered Hebrews 10:7, where the writer spoke of Jesus saying, "Behold, I have come, in the volume of the Book it is written of Me," referring to the Old Testament prophesies about His coming, suffering, death, resurrection and return to heaven, and the New Testament writings fulfilling them.

I had studied the entire Bible at both of our churches, and I realized how much I missed it and how easily its void had spun my life around, becoming a person neither my husband nor I liked very much.

So, consumed with the guilt of leaving my First Love, Jesus, and fearful I'd ventured too far away to return, I cried out, pleading with Him to embrace me again. I began a desperate quest to reignite my love for Him through His Word and asked if He would help me find Bible study resources. He, in His faithfulness and lovingkindness, accommodated me in a special way, leading me to an online Torah class which provided in-depth Bible teachings on the Old and New Testaments, bringing Yeshua to life on practically every page. Studying His Word had become more exciting to me than ever before and, unknowingly, prepared me for such a time as this.

I gradually drew closer and closer to Him, becoming sensitive again to His presence in my life, His strength during my weakness, His comfort during my pain, His peace during my anxiety, His patience during my frustration, and His promise in Isaiah 46:3-4, where He said, "You....who have been upheld by Me from birth, who have been carried from the womb: even to your old age, I am He - And even to gray hairs I will carry you. I have made, and I will bear; even I will carry, and will deliver you."

I needed the Lord to carry Euvon and me now; so, while he slept under the watchful eye of the anesthesiologist, trusting his jugular vein to the hand of God, I read His Word, the Word He esteems above His very Name (Psalm 138:2), and received comfort and peace, knowing nothing would happen to my husband without God's permission.

I finished my meal and returned to the hospital, finding Euvon awake and starving. I could see the protrusion along his neck where the catheter line had been placed. The bandage on the right side of his chest covered the catheter, but the lumens were also visible. Euvon was nauseated, yet concerned about eating something nutritious; so, I returned to the cafe I'd just left and selected a few items I knew he could enjoy and yet would be healthy for him, as well. The meal helped his nausea subside enough for him to go home.

As she prepared his discharge papers and instructions, the nurse asked him why he needed the catheter. He told her about his overall condition and how excited he was to soon be undergoing the immunotherapy, which he explained in as much detail as he could understand. When she expressed her sympathy, he gave God glory for his journey. We introduced her to our Savior because in the midst of this diagnosis, He had drawn us closer to Him and to each other.

We were being weaned out of our old lifestyle, and Euvon proudly announced that in one more year, when he turned sixty-two, he was going to retire. Hallelujah! Before this diagnosis, he had planned to work until he could no longer walk or breathe. But now, he was finally ready to set his tools down and enjoy his life and family.

There were many hidden things that belonged to God, including the fullness of our days. But those things He revealed to us, including stage IV prostate cancer, gave us the wisdom to know the importance of enjoying whatever remaining years He graced us with together. We were confident our lives were in His hands, which excited us to see where He would lead us beyond retirement.

We gave the nurse a hug and left hoping she understood how much she needed the Lord, His love, forgiveness, and redemption, in Yeshua's Name.

Clinical Trial: involves the patient in medical research studies. jmj

Chapter Twenty-eight

IMMUNOTHERAPY

With the catheter now in place, we were ready to begin the Provenge immunotherapy. Euvon was scheduled to receive the first treatment within the next two Tuesdays, which was the day following the Presidential Inauguration.

On Inaugural Day, I prepared as many meals and snacks as possible, since he wouldn't be able to eat eight hours before nor drink anything four hours before the treatment. He figured if he stuffed himself while he could, he'd still be full the next day.

But, while we celebrated the inauguration of our president, an unsettling feeling stuck in the back of my throat. I'd lost my nerve to go with my husband to the treatment center. Hospitals, needles, extractions, and infusions had become too much for me. While I didn't want him to go alone, I'd grown tired of seeing him at the mercy of others, and I needed a mental break. I knew I had no right to feel that way because he was the one standing central in the crossfire. But, I did. And to be honest, I also felt scared.

So, just before bedtime, I found the courage to tell him I didn't want to go with him. He understood, certain he'd be okay going alone. He took the news so well, I felt more guilty than ever, and after he went to sleep, I called our daughter, Cristina. It was too late for her to come for his leukapheresis procedure, but she promised she would come down from New York and accompany him to the hospital for his infusion.

Euvon arrived promptly at 7:00 on Tuesday morning for his first leukapheresis session, where two attendants met him at the door, matched his ID with theirs, settled him in a man-cave recliner, and connected the tubes from the machine to the catheter extending from his chest. Most of his torso was covered with sensors and probes.

Midway through the procedure, Euvon called me, briefly complaining that he was getting chills and feeling tingly. But he also sounded grateful he was being well taken care of, and the staff was doing everything they could to make him comfortable. One of the attendants kept him covered him with blankets and fed him several anti-acids to keep him from getting heartburn, while another attendant tuned in to a jazz station to help him relax. Things moved along relatively well, and he was able to take short naps.

Once the treatment was complete, the attendants cleaned, sanitized, and sealed the catheter ports. Satisfied, yet tired, he looked forward to going home and resting for the evening.

Cris arrived on Thursday, and the following day accompanied him to the hospital for his first Provenge infusion. She was happy she'd been able to go so she could see exactly how it was done. She also felt comfortable about him receiving the next two series of treatments alone.

Euvon, too, was so convinced the second treatment would replicate the first, he didn't think I needed to accompany him, thank God. In fact, he decided to go to work before going to his 7:00 a.m. appointment.

During the second leukapheresis procedure, he felt the same chills. But then, he also felt woozy and fearful that one of his knees might give out. He was given anti-acids again to ward off heartburn, and when he came home, he ate dinner and went directly to bed.

After the infusion three days later, he developed flu-like symptoms; the stuffy nose and chest congestion, with muscle and groin pain. But he stood like a champ, taking hot showers to soothe his bones and waking up to another work day.

With one more series to go, we were getting excited, realizing we'd be done by spring, which was fast approaching.

The final treatment was more intense and harsh than Euvon had anticipated. He had trouble with excessive rigors and nagging groin pain. He came home more tired and woozy than in the past, and I wished that I'd gone with him. But, he said the attendants were constantly by his side, keeping him warm with blankets and watching over him like an eagle over her young, all the while keeping the jazz music flowing. He didn't want anyone there to know, but he'd become extremely weak at one point and could barely focus, unsure if he'd be able to drive himself home after the session.

Apparently, signs of weakness were obvious because once the treatment was complete, he was encouraged to drink orange, cranberry, or grape juice, and munch on a snack so he'd be strong enough to drive. He settled on two bottles of water and pretzels, not wanting to drink anything with sugar, since he felt his body was vulnerable at that point.

The attendants continued hovering over and pampering him, asking again and again, "Are you okay?" They wanted to make sure he was fully able to drive safely home.

Regardless of how he felt, "Yes," was his interminable response, because he just wanted to get home, take a long, hot shower, nourish himself, and rest.

"I will restore you to health and heal your wounds," declares the Lord.
Jeremiah 30:17

Jesus went through all the towns and villages....healing every disease and sickness.
Matthew 9:35

Chapter Twenty-nine

RECOVERY

While this tired, worn out man replenished his body with baked sockeye salmon, roasted sweet potato, and steamed broccoli, I helped myself to a heavy dose of guilt.

It didn't matter that we had no idea this final phase would be his most traumatic and frightening ordeal. Although he admitted he'd tried hard to ignore it with sleep, except for a few short intervals, he was practically awake the entire time.

I apologized for not being with him, but never one to make another feel regretful, he brushed it off with a, "But the Lord was there," and, "Hey, I was okay. There was nothing you could have done. Everybody watched me like a hawk and pawed over me like a puppy," and, "I'm just glad it's all over, and you were here to make this wonderful dinner for me, 'cause I was starving."

His encouragement sorta kinda worked. I mean, who could have surpassed the Lord being with him? Certainly not I. Who could've hovered over him better than the experts, who probably would've pushed me aside to accommodate him at a moment's notice? Never not I. And who could've possibly cared for and nourished him post-procedure at home more efficiently than I? No one. Realizing we were all at our assigned posts, I felt somewhat better already.

That Friday, he returned to Georgetown Hospital for his final infusion. Then he had one last appointment to return to the hospital a few days later to extract that menacing catheter, and we couldn't wait.

But again, what we thought would be a quick catheter removal and return to work was quite the opposite. We'd forgotten it ran through his jugular vein and just couldn't be yanked out. Euvon would have to be anesthetized again. Alone. He had planned to go to work after the procedure; so, he'd left home without me.

He called me just before surgery, disturbed by this turn of events. I offered to come to the hospital and take him home after the catheter was removed. We could return for his truck at another time. He refused, insisting instead to just get it done and be gone for good. He promised, though, that he wouldn't rush his recovery. He wouldn't leave until he was certain he was completely ready, with steady hands and feet.

Time crawled while I busied myself with minutiae until late evening when he finally walked in. We whewed and glory hallelujahed because his entire immunotherapy process had finally come to a close. We reflected on the last six or so weeks, thankful that Euvon had been graced, again, with few side effects.

And, although our emotions fluctuated consistently, our general routine had not. Except for the three Tuesdays he had to be available for the cell collection, my husband had not missed a day from work nor a Sunday from church. His appetite remained healthy, we continued visiting loved ones, we enjoyed our time together, planned his retirement, and almost every day ended with peaceful sleep.

After a day or two, Euvon took a mental note of that six-week immunotherapy schedule. Monday, work; Tuesday, cell collection; Wednesday and Thursday, work; Friday, infusion and work; Saturday, rest; Sunday, church and rest; Monday, work and at the hospital to sanitize his catheter; Tuesday, work; Wednesday, work and at the hospital to sanitize the catheter. Thursday, work; Friday, work and at the hospital to sanitize the catheter. This cycle repeated at two additional intervals.

We prayed the immunotherapy itself would be a success. We would find out in a couple of weeks.

Chapter Thirty

REGRESSED PROGRESSION

"Heaven help us! Lord, have mercy," we anguished on our pillows. What did we miss? Where did we go wrong?

Euvon's psa count had climbed again, and it had only been a couple of weeks since the final Provenge therapy. That fast. The scar on his chest from the catheter was still healing. He showed no visible signs that something was amiss, but I was an emotional and spiritual mess, dazed and confused. All I felt was the clash of my internal organs. My love for the Lord was steadfast, but my faith took a nose-dive, and I didn't know what to think.

Doctor Dawson, however, never flinched at the news, and neither did Euvon. He stayed with the, "So, what's next?" attitude. In spite of the depth of the diagnosis and the intensity of his treatments, he maintained faith and joy, trusting each therapy to advance him toward healing's end.

Another hormone therapy pill called Xtandi, four of which he would begin taking daily, was added to his regimen, which the doctor explained had already been planned once the Provenge treatments were completed. Although his psa level had increased again, the immunotherapy would probably kickstart with Xtandi. Euvon asked how long he would have to take the medicine, to which she replied, "Until it stops working. If all goes well, for the rest of your life."

The first delivery of the medicine which would, thereafter, occur on a monthly basis, was accompanied by a small book listing a plethora of possible side effects and remedies, if needed. It also included a small sign to post on our front door in case Euvon was too slow to answer and sign for the medicine. He was given ID to present in case he became debilitated in public. I rebuked all that thoughtfulness.

The pharmacy systematically called two weeks after each prescription to ensure the next refill arrived well before he ran out. They always asked if he had any problems and told us they would be available if he needed counsel. It felt good knowing there was some concern from his entire medical team.

Well, bless the Lord, oh my soul, the only problems Euvon had were fatigue and minor joint pains, although we weren't sure if they were from the medicine or the disease. Even though he had decreased his hours significantly, his job still kept him stressful, and he'd often come home worn and achy. His energy and health levels may have been better had he been retired, but that was not yet the case. I noticed, however, when he rested on Saturdays, he was more active the next day, and physically prepared for his Monday, back-to-work schedule.

The Trial of Stage IV Prostate Cancer

PART SIX

THE VERDICT

In all these things we are more than
conquerors through Him who loved us.
For I am convinced that neither death
nor life, neither angels nor demons,
neither the present nor the future, nor
any powers, neither height nor depth,
nor anything else in all creation will be
able to separate us from the love of God
that is in Christ Jesus our Lord.
Romans 8:37-39

Chapter Thirty-one

A WIN-WIN CONDITION

As summer eased peacefully in, Euvon's psa count slowly declined again until it became undetectable. For the first time in a long, drawn out while, we felt as though we could breathe again. We took several short vacations and entertained our children and grandchildren, which had become of even greater importance to us and truly cherished times.

Autumn's leaves gradually transitioned into warm earth tones before drifting to the ground, occasionally blanketed under the winter's snow.

Euvon finally turned sixty-two, and feeling himself transitioning, decided to retire. He'd begun to tire more easily, and the aches had become more prominent. He wanted to hang up his hat, throw away his boots, and rest.

These past few years have motivated us to peek into Apostle Paul's declarations sprinkled throughout Second Corinthians four and six, where he summarized his ministry and life as "hard-pressed on every side, yet not crushed; we are perplexed, but not in despair; persecuted, but not forsaken; struck down, but not destroyed; as dying, yet behold, we live; chastened, and yet not killed; as sorrowful, yet always rejoicing."

I was reminded of the Lord carrying Ezekiel, in Chapter thirty-seven, down in the midst of a valley of dry bones, and asking him, "Can these bones live?" to which Ezekiel answered, "O Lord God, You know."

God Almighty then instructed Ezekiel to prophesy upon those bones, and say to them, 'O you dry bones, hear the word of the Lord. Thus says the Lord God to these bones: Surely, I will cause breath to enter into you and you shall live. I will put sinews on you and will bring flesh upon you, cover you with skin and put breath in you, and you shall live. Then you shall know that I am the Lord.'

And, that's been our prayer, that the Lord would speak to Euvon's bones and breathe healing upon them. We've prayed fervently, too, for Him to remove all sickness and disease from us, from our children, and from our children's children forever.

Chapter Thirty-two

AMEN

Almost two years since the immunotherapy and one year post retirement, we continue to stand face to face against a formidable foe. Nonetheless, Euvon is thriving well, and our romance and intimacy remain active and strong.

He continues his scheduled monthly visits with his doctor for blood work and consultation, and maintains his daily Xtandi dose and the trimonthly hormone-shot routine. The monthly calcium shot has been temporarily replaced with antibiotics due to a cancer related gum infection that has impacted his jaw bone, but has failed to diminish his appetite, praise God.

We are involved in a low impact exercise program, and walking and swimming as often as we can has kept our bodies limber and oxygenated.

We trust that the Lord is still in the process of healing Euvon His way while we cling to and wait on Him.

Our medical team and we are generals and captains, but God Almighty is our Commander-in-Chief. Sometimes He instructs Euvon and me as He did Jehoshaphat and the people of Judah in Second Chronicles 20:15, when several pagan tribes rose up against them, to "Be not dismayed by reason of this great multitude, for the battle is not yours, but God's."

There are other times when He instructs us as He did Joshua, who prepared to engage in his first war in the Promised Land against the city of Jericho. In Joshua 6:1-5, The Lord told him to gather his warriors and walk silently around Jericho's walls six days. Then on the seventh day, they were to march around the city seven times, and when the trumpets sounded, they were to shout. The walls would fall, they would defeat the inhabitants.

Through this particular time in our lives, we believe we've been given a combination of both instructions, at times to be still and see God move on our behalf, and at other times to work and march out our faith with a shout of praise.

In the meantime, wherever life takes us and however bumpy the ride, may we travel fearlessly, hopeful, trusting that Abba, Father, our Great Physician and Healer, will one day guide us safely Home, in Yeshua's Name. Amen.

The Trial of Stage IV Prostate Cancer

PART SEVEN

Lessons Gleaned Along The Way

His Word is in my heart as a burning fire shut up in my bones.

Jeremiah 20:9

HEALING SCRIPTURES POSTED ON OUR WALLS

JEHOVAH RAPHA, OUR HEALER

I WILL PUT NONE OF THESE DISEASES ON YOU….FOR I AM THE LORD WHO HEALS YOU.
EXODUS 15:26

AND AS YOUR DAYS, SO SHALL YOUR STRENGTH BE.
DEUT. 33:25

I HAVE HEARD YOUR PRAYER, I HAVE SEEN YOUR TEARS: SURELY I WILL HEAL YOU.
2 KINGS 20:5

BLESS THE LORD, O MY SOUL...WHO FORGIVES ALL YOUR INIQUITIES, WHO HEALS ALL YOUR DISEASES. PSALM. 103:3

HE SENT HIS WORD, AND HEALED THEM, AND DELIVERED THEM FROM THEIR DESTRUCTION. PSALM. 107:20

I WILL ATTEND TO THE WORD OF GOD. I WILL NOT LET THE WORD DEPART FROM MY EYES. I WILL KEEP THE WORD IN THE MIDST OF MY MIND. FOR IT IS LIFE TO ME AND HEALTH TO ALL MY FLESH.(PARAPHRASED) PROVERBS 4:20-22

BY HIS STRIPES, WE ARE HEALED.
ISAIAH 53:5

I WILL RESTORE HEALTH TO YOU, AND HEAL YOU OF YOUR WOUNDS. JEREMIAH 30:17

JESUS WILL COME AND HEAL ME. (PARAPHRASED) MATTHEW 8:7

DAUGHTER (SON), BE OF GOOD COMFORT; YOUR FAITH HAS MADE YOU WHOLE. MATTHEW 9:22

PRECIOUS FAITH; PRECIOUS BLOOD; PRECIOUS PROMISES. I PET. 1:19; II PET. I:1, 4

In YESHUA'S Name, Amen

UNHEALTHY FOODS WE AVOID

Transfats, including lard, margarine, corn oil, vegetable oil, soybean oil, palm oil, cottonseed oil, sunflower oil, and safflower oil.

Pork

Processed foods, including hot dogs, sausage, bacon, pepperoni, and lunchmeat. On rare occasions, we will enjoy organic hotdogs with organic hotdog buns, organic lunchmeat, and organic turkey bacon and sausage.

Pesticide-laden commercial salad bars.

Excessive amounts of:

High-fat dairy foods

Pickled, preserved, or salted foods

Smoked meats

Foods fried in high heat

Broiled, overdone meat

Charcoal-grilled meat

Red meat. (We occasionally eat organic beef and lamb).

HEALTHY FOODS WE'VE INVESTED IN

ORGANIC

Strawberries
Blueberries
Raspberries
Blackberries
Cherries
Imported Grapes
Tangerines
Nectarines
Pears
Peaches
Plums
All Leafy Green Vegetables
Cucumbers

Carrots
All lettuce
Most Root Vegetables
Winter Squash
Summer Squash
Green Onions
Beef (can buy grass-fed)
Lamb (can buy grass-fed)
Poultry

CONVENTIONAL

Grapefruit
Mangoes
Cantaloupes
Watermelons
Bananas
Pineapples
Honeydew Melons
Coconut
Papayas
Lemons
Limes
All Cabbage Family Vegetables

Asparagus
Broccoli
Cauliflower
Sweet Potatoes/Yams
Mushrooms
Non-GMO Corn
Avocados
Onions
Garlic

Fish (sockeye salmon, king salmon, keta salmon, hake, rainbow trout, dover sole, sardines, herring, haddock, and whiting)

BREAKFASTS EUVON HAS ENJOYED

No specific time is given for doneness, since every stove is different.

We've discarded our microwave, since Euvon has already been exposed to regular x-rays and scans. Our nonstick cookware have also been thrown out because they contain toxins that can leach into our food. Instead, we cook with stainless steel, ceramic, and non-porous stoneware. We've also returned to the old fashioned way of cooking and reheating food - the good ole stovetop and conventional oven, along with the occasional use of a countertop rotisserie or glass enclosed convection oven.

Since this is not a cookbook, and I rarely measure, most of these recipes give approximate ingredient measurements; therefore, if any of them is appealing to try, the palette's imagination should be at work. Have fun and enjoy.

Egg Omelet and Toast

Organic olive oil, enough to cover bottom of pan

2 teaspoons each, onion, organic red pepper, organic tomato, organic mushrooms, chopped

2 organic eggs, beaten

Grey salt or sea salt, pepper to taste

2 slices organic wheat or whole grain bread

2 teaspoons organic ghee

Heat oil in medium pan on low until hot. Saute onion, pepper, tomato, and mushrooms until tender. Pour in eggs and let set on bottom. Fold in half and cover for thirty seconds. Turn over and cover for an additional thirty seconds or until completely done. If preparing an omelet is too time-consuming, simply add eggs to sauteed vegetables and scramble till cooked through. Salt and pepper to taste. Remove.

Toast bread until lightly brown. Spread with ghee, and enjoy.

Sauteed Apples

Organic olive oil or organic coconut oil

2 organic granny smith apples

2 organic gala apples

2 organic fuji apples

2 organic red delicious apples

2 teaspoons organic ghee

2 teaspoons organic maple syrup (optional)

Cinnamon, nutmeg, vanilla to taste

Heat oil in pan on low until hot. Peel apples halfway and slice. If peeled completely, applesauce will result, which is fine. Add apples to hot oil, cover, and saute till tender. Add maple syrup if additional sweetness is desired. Add cinnamon, nutmeg, and vanilla to taste.

Pancakes

2 cups organic all purpose, whole wheat, or buckwheat flour

5 teaspoons baking powder

1/2 teaspoon sea salt

2 cups goat milk or organic unsweetened almond milk

2 organic eggs, beaten

3 tablespoons organic olive oil

Cinnamon and vanilla to taste

Enough oil to make pancakes

Organic ghee

Organic maple syrup

Organic olive oil for pan

Combine dry ingredients. Blend in 1 cup of milk, eggs, and oil. Add additional milk until desired batter consistency. Add cinnamon and vanilla to taste. Heat oil in pan on medium-low till hot. Pour ¼ cup pancake mix into pan and cook till lightly brown. Turn over and cook until brown. Remove from pan and spread with ghee. Top with syrup or warmed fruit.

Fruit Topping

2 cups organic fresh or frozen berries
1/2 to 1 cup filtered water
1 tablespoon organic cornstarch
3 tablespoons filtered water

In medium saucepan, bring water and berries to a boil. Lower heat to a simmer. Mix cornstarch with remaining water until smooth. Slowly add to fruit until thickened to desired consistency. Simmer about an additional minute and remove from heat.

French Toast

Organic olive oil
Organic ghee
6 slices organic whole wheat, french, or spelt bread
3 organic eggs
1 cup goat milk or organic almond milk
1/2 cup organic whipping cream (on rare occasions)
1/2 teaspoon cinnamon
1/2 teaspoon nutmeg

Pinch sea salt
1 teaspoon vanilla
Organic maple syrup or organic fruit topping
Beat eggs and milk. Add cinnamon, nutmeg, vanilla, and sea salt. Heat pan on medium. Add equal amounts of ghee and olive oil to fill bottom of pan. Dip slice of bread in egg mixture and place in pan. When golden brown, turn over and cook until done. Top with syrup or fruit sauce.

Organic Grits
4-½ cups water
1 cup grits
1 teaspoon sea salt
4 teaspoons organic ghee
Pour water into medium saucepan and bring to boil. Lower heat and slowly stir in grits. Stir consistently to prevent lumps from forming. Simmer till smooth in texture. Add salt and ghee to taste.

Organic Oatmeal
4 cups water
1 cup organic old fashioned oatmeal
1 cup organic instant oatmeal
1 tablespoon organic ghee
2 tablespoons organic maple syrup

Salt, cinnamon to taste
Pour water into medium saucepan and bring to boil. Lower heat and slowly stir in old fashioned oatmeal. Simmer approximately 10 minutes. Add instant oatmeal and simmer another 5 minutes. Stir in ghee, maple syrup, and cinnamon.

Fresh Organic Fruit Breakfast

2 tablespoons each, strawberries, blueberries, cherries
1/2 cup goat milk, whole milk, or organic Greek yogurt
1 teaspoon walnuts
1 teaspoon unsweetened coconut, shredded
2 teaspoons organic dark chocolate bits, chopped
2 teaspoons raisins
1 teaspoon currants
Mix fruit in bowl. Top with yogurt and optional toppings.

LUNCHES EUVON HAS ENJOYED

Mediterranean Salad

2 cups organic romaine and baby romaine lettuce

1/2 organic cucumber, sliced

10 organic grape or cherry tomatoes, sliced

1/4 cup cooked organic quinoa

1/4 cup red onion, sliced

1/2 cup organic kalamata olives

1/4 cup organic feta cheese (on rare occasions)

1/4 cup organic broccoli sprouts

Dressing

1/2 cup organic Abba's (olive) oil

3 tablespoons balsamic vinegar or Braggs apple cider vinegar

1 tablespoon fresh lemon juice

1 tablespoon local or organic raw honey
1or 2 cloves garlic, crushed
Himalayan pink sea salt, pepper to taste
Mix all ingredients

Salmon Salad

1 pound sockeye-salmon, poached, baked, or sauteed
3 cups organic vegetable stock or water
3 tablespoons organic Abba's oil
1 tablespoon organic ghee
1/2 small onion, chopped
1 stalk organic celery, chopped
1/2 teaspoon organic tumeric powder
1/2 teaspoon garlic powder
1/2 cup or less organic mayonnaise
1/4 cup or less goat or sheep yogurt

Poach salmon in broth or water. If baking or sautéing salmon, place in pan with oil and ghee. Remove when done and extract any small bones. Mash with fork and add remaining ingredients. Serve with salad or a slice of organic bread.

Organic Kale-Carrot Salad

1 pound fresh organic kale, finely chopped

2 organic carrots, finely chopped

3 tablespoons - 1/4 cup Braggs amino acids

1/4 cup nutritional yeast

1/2 medium red onion, chopped

2 cloves garlic, minced

1/3 cup organic Abba's oil

1/4 cup lemon juice

1/4 cup toasted organic sesame seeds, sunflower seeds, and chopped cashews

Blend all ingredients in a bowl, adjust taste, and let sit or refrigerate for about two hours before serving.

Cooked Quinoa

1 cup organic quinoa

Organic Abba's oil

1 cup chicken stock

1 cup water

1/2 teaspoon organic tumeric

1/2 teaspoon each, organic basil, sage, oregano, thyme, rosemary, crushed

Sea salt, pepper to taste

Saute quinoa in oil approximately 5 minutes. Add chicken stock and simmer about 15 to 20 minutes, until soft and flaky. Season with tumeric, sea salt, and pepper. Add crushed herbs and fluff. Add to salad or serve as a side dish to chicken, fish, or lamb.

Baked Cod Fish Cakes

1 pound cod fish, shredded in blender or food processor
1/2 small onion, crushed
1 stalk organic celery, crushed
1 organic egg, beaten
1/4 teaspoon organic mustard seed
1/2 teaspoon organic tumeric powder
Sea salt, pepper to taste
Add shredded fish and all other ingredients to bowl. Shape into patties and bake on 350 degrees about 10 to 15 minutes.
Serve with organic crackers and salad.

Vegetable Smoothie

1 cup frozen organic kale
1small organic carrot, finely chopped
1 cup savoy or red cabbage, or brussel sprouts, shredded
1 teaspoon psyllium
1/2 cucumber, sliced thin
1/2 organic red delicious apple, chopped
1 cup water

1 cup crushed ice

Blend all ingredients and enjoy.

Fruit Smoothie

1/2 cup each, frozen organic blueberries, raspberries, strawberries, blackberries, cherries, and grapes

2 tablespoons organic oat bran

1 teaspoon psyllium

1 tablespoon ground organic coconut

1 tablespoon ground organic chocolate

2 tablespoons organic tart cherry juice concentrate

1/2 teaspoon vitamin C powder

1/2 cup water

1/2 cup crushed ice

Blend all ingredients and add additional water for the desired consistency.

DINNERS EUVON HAS ENJOYED

That Infamous Chicken Soup

1 or 2 cups of organic chicken breast, cubed

Organic Abba's oil

1 small onion, cubed

2 cloves garlic, minced

2 stalks organic celery, cubed

2 organic carrots, cubed

2 organic tomatoes, chopped

4 cups organic chicken stock

2 cups water

Celtic salt, pepper, tumeric

organic thyme

organic cilantro

Saute garlic, onion, celery, carrots, and chicken in oil on low. Add chicken stock and water. Bring to boil. Cover and simmer for a few minutes. Add tomatoes and continue to simmer till tomatoes are tender. Season with celtic salt, pepper, turmeric, thyme, and cilantro at the end of cooking. Toast a slice of organic whole wheat bread and spread with homemade ghee.

Sauteed Sockeye Salmon

Organic olive oil
Organic ghee
8 oz sockeye salmon (or other low mercury wild Pacific fish)
Fresh lemon juice
1/2 onion, sliced
2 or 3 cloves garlic, sliced
1/4 organic bell pepper, sliced
1/2 stalk organic celery, sliced
1/2 cup organic tomatoes, sliced
1/4 cup fresh fennel bulb, chopped
1/4 teaspoon each, fresh organic thyme, rosemary, oregano, and marjoram
seafood seasoning
tumeric
Sea salt, and pepper to taste

Add equal amounts of ghee and olive oil to cover bottom of pan. Place salmon in the middle of the pan; surround and top with sliced vegetables and herbs. Drizzle all ingredients with lemon juice, olive oil, and melted ghee. Add salt, pepper, tumeric, and seafood seasoning to taste. Cover and saute on low until done. Serve with roasted sweet potato and sauteed kale, cabbage, spinach, or brussel sprouts.

Sauteed Lamb

1 organic or grass-fed lamb chop or shoulder blade
Sea salt, pepper
Organic tumeric
1/2 cup onion, chopped
3 cloves garlic, sliced
1 carrot, sliced thin
1/2 cup cabbage, shredded
Organic Abba's oil
Organic ghee
Fresh organic thyme leaves
Fresh organic mint leaves

Season with salt, pepper, and tumeric. Pour enough oil and ghee to cover bottom of pan. Place lamb in middle of pan; surround and top with onion, garlic, carrot, cabbage, and herbs. Season vegetables lightly with additional salt, pepper, and tumeric. Saute lamb and vegetables until lamb is browned on one side. Turn over and cook on other side. Adjust vegetables around and on top of lamb. Once lamb is brown, remove from pan if desired doneness is reached. If not, turn off heat and cover for a few minutes.

Baked Chicken Wings

Preheat oven to 350 degrees. Use same ingredients and instructions as Sauteed Sockeye Salmon. Omit fennel and seafood seasoning. Bake in glass dish until done.

Dry Brined Whole Rotisserie Chicken

Dry Brine Mix:

1/2 cup Mediterranean kosher sea salt
2 tablespoons black peppercorns
1-2 teaspoons organic garlic powder
1-2 teaspoons organic celery seeds
1 tablespoon organic thyme
1 tablespoon organic rosemary
1 tablespoon organic lemon zest
2 teaspoons organic orange zest
2 teaspoons organic tumeric
1 teaspoon paprika

Chicken Rub

1 tablespoon organic Abba's oil

1 tablespoon organic ghee

1 tablespoon local or organic honey

1 teaspoon organic mustard

1 teaspoon salt

1 teaspoon pepper

Two days before, grind all dry brine ingredients together. Rub chicken in oil. Rub brine over chicken, one tablespoon at a time, until evenly spread. Lift breast skin and rub directly on breast meat. Place in glass or stainless steel dish, cover, and refrigerate overnight. Turn chicken over on its breast and refrigerate a second night.

On the day of cooking, let chicken sit at room temperature at least four hours. Rinse, and pat dry. Mix Rub and lightly spread over chicken. Rotisserie chicken according to directions, or bake on 350 degrees until done.

Lentil Soup (May also substitute any bean, but cooking times will vary)

1 medium onion, chopped

2 stalks organic celery, chopped

3 cloves garlic, minced

3 tablespoons organic Abba's oil

3 cups organic chicken stock

2 cups water
2 cups lentils
2 organic carrots, cubed
2-3 organic tomatoes, chopped
1 teaspoon organic tumeric
1/2 teaspoon cumin
1/2 teaspoon coriander
Salt flakes, pepper, to taste
Saute onion, celery, and garlic in Abba's oil to release flavor, approximately 2 minutes. Add at least 3 cups chicken stock, 2 cups water, lentils, and carrots. Simmer until lentils are almost tender. Add tumeric, cumin, coriander, and tomatoes. Cook till tender. Salt and pepper to taste.

Curry Rice

2 cups water
1 cup organic basmati rice
3 tablespoons organic coconut oil
1 small onion, chopped
1 clove garlic, minced
3 tablespoons curry powder
2 cups organic chicken broth or water
1 cup organic carrots, thinly sliced
1/2 cup organic red potatoes, cubed (optional)

1/2 - 1 cup organic coconut milk or organic raw coconut water

Salt and pepper to taste

Cook rice according to instructions. Melt coconut oil in medium saucepan. Saute onion and garlic on low till translucent. Stir in curry powder. Slowly stir in broth or water. Bring to boil. Lower heat to simmer. Add carrots and potatoes and cook till tender. Add desired additional curry powder. Salt and pepper to taste. Pour over rice and enjoy. May also add meat or fish.

Mashed Cauliflower

1 head cauliflower

2-3 cups organic chicken or vegetable broth

1/2 small onion, crushed

2 cloves garlic, crushed

1 tablespoon organic ghee

Salt and pepper to taste

In a pot, bring broth to a boil. Add cauliflower, onion, and garlic and simmer for about fifteen minutes. Remove from heat and mash. Season with organic ghee, salt and pepper.

Asparagus Soup

2 pounds fresh asparagus

1 onion, chopped

4 cloves garlic, sliced

2 stalks organic celery, sliced

1/2 organic green pepper, chopped

1 cup organic mushrooms, chopped

Organic Abba's oil

5 - 6 cups organic chicken or vegetable stock

1 tablespoon organic tumeric

Sea salt, pepper to taste

Saute all ingredients in Abba's oil approximately ten minutes, stirring constantly. Add stock, cover and simmer fifteen to twenty minutes. Remove from stove and let cool. Then, blend in batches in blender or food processor. Return to pot and heat, adding desired amount of sea salt, pepper, and tumeric.

Baked French Fries

3 organic russet, golden, or red potatoes, cut in strips

Organic Abba's oil

Sea salt, pepper

Place unbleached parchment paper on baking sheet. Toss potato strips in oil and lay flat on parchment paper. Sprinkle with salt and pepper and bake on 350 degrees, turning once or twice. Remove from oven and serve.

Baked Sweet Potato Fries

2 Yams, cut in strips
Organic Coconut Oil
Sea Salt
Cinnamon

Place unbleached parchment paper on baking sheet. Toss yams in oil and lay flat on parchment paper. Sprinkle with salt and cinnamon and bake on 375 degrees, turning once or twice. Remove from oven and serve.

Ghee

1 pound organic butter
2-quart saucepan
Gauze or cheesecloth
Strainer
Glass container

Melt butter in saucepan on medium until white milk fat settles on top, 10 to 15 minutes.

Let cool slightly. Fold gauze or cheesecloth into four layers. Set inside strainer and pour clear golden ghee through strainer into container.

Ghee may be kept at room temperature indefinitely, as long as no other moisture or food comes in contact with it. Wipe utensil clean after each serving.

Date Puree

2 cups dates

Water

Place dates in a large bowl and add enough water to cover about one inch above top layer. Cover and let sit approximately eight hours or overnight, until softened. Blend dates in food processor or blender, adding one tablespoon of water at a time until date puree is at desired consistency.

Dates are nutritional and may be used in place of sugar. Retain and refrigerate the date liquid for use as an additional sweetener. Spread date puree on natural wax paper or unbleached parchment paper, fold, and freeze. Break a piece when needed to sweeten food or drink. Otherwise, it will last about a week in the refrigerator.

ESSENTIAL AND CARRIER OILS WE USE

Extensive research and consulting with a medical expert is strongly recommended before using any of these oils, which may react differently with each person. I am no expert in the use of essential oils and, therefore, hold myself harmless of any negative reaction.

Cinnamon Cassia - Mentioned in the Bible. It is good for viral and bacterial infections, nail fungus, and arthritis.

Clove - Good for tooth, gum, and throat pain, indigestion, and nausea. Helps treat wounds, mouth ulcers, insect bites, stings, and headaches. It also helps anti-aging, increases blood flow and circulation.

Eucalyptus - Can be used as a decongestant or deodorant. Treats wounds, cuts, insect bites, stings, and is good as a sore throat gargle. Helps muscle pain from sprained ligaments, pain, and rheumatism. Effective against cavities, plaque, and gingivitis. It also increases circulation. Use sparingly with carrier oil.

Frankincense - Gifted to Christ at birth. Can help toothaches. Tightens skin. Helps remove surgical scars when applied topically; promotes regeneration of healthy cells, tones and tightens under eye area, helps insomnia when massaged into temples. Great room freshener when added to pure water and/or vodka.

Helichrysum - Helps clear boils, skin spots, rashes, and pimples. Can be applied topically to cuts and wounds. Helps arthritis. Helps detox the liver when applied to the bottom of feet. Prevents dehydration, and helps surgical scars fade. Blends well with lavender and frankincense.

Hyssop - Referred to in the Bible. Helps with gums, muscles, limbs; improves circulation, rheumatoid arthritis, gout, and swelling. Add three to five drops in a diffuser diluted with water and inhale. Or add the drops to a cotton ball moist with a carrier oil, such as Abba's oil, coconut oil, or castor oil and apply to skin.

Lavender - Promotes sleep, decreases anxiety, helps acne, muscle pain, and joints. Apply on skin with carrier oil.

Lemon - Conditions hair and skin when used with jojoba or sweet almond oil. Helps gout. Cleanses the liver and kidneys. Add to bath or apply to skin with carrier oil.

Myrrh - Gift presented to Baby Yeshua. Immune system builder; helps joint pain, indigestion, cough, anti-aging; promotes healthy skin, aids gum care, prevents hair loss, helps against colds, helps keep body free of toxins, and heals wounds. Blends well with frankincense, lavender, sandalwood, and tea tree.

Orange - Helps the immune system, inflammation, eliminates toxins, helps anxiety, good for skin and relaxing muscles. Blends well with cinnamon, clove, frankincense, and sandalwood.

Peppermint - Aids indigestion, headache, fever, relieves Irritable Bowel Syndrome, abdominal pain, urinary tract infections, and helps gums remove germs. Helps headaches when applied on forehead with carrier oil. Soothes nausea when inhaled. Helps respiratory issues and boosts the immune system, helps against bacterial strains, and stimulates hair growth. Blends well with eucalyptus and lemon.

Sandalwood - Mentioned in the Bible. Anti-inflammatory. Protects wounds, boils, and pimples from infections. Helps digestion, circulation, cramps, gums, strengthens muscles, tightens skin, helps scars heal, disinfects, and helps internal infections, such as throat, stomach, and intestines. Treats coughs, helps with anxiety, and can be used as a deodorant ingredient. Soothes skin when mixed with a carrier oil, such as Abba's oil, coconut oil, or castor oil. Mixes well with lavender, myrrh, rose, and ylang-ylang.

Tea Tree - Treats bacterial infections in colon, stomach, and intestines. Helps colds, flu, and clears marks from boils and acne. Helps nail fungus and muscle pain. Add diluted to scalp to prevent hair loss. Acts as insect repellant. Can be applied to wounds, insect bites, and stings. Boosts the immune system. Blends well with cinnamon, clove, lemon, and myrrh.

Texas cedarwood - Cedar wood is mentioned in the Bible. Good for eczema, wounds, muscle aches, and toothaches. Helps release toxins, stimulates the metabolism and tones muscles. Aids the liver, kidneys, digestive and lymphatic systems, gout, rheumatism, and arthritis. Helps colds, coughs, and phlegm. Repels insects. Blends well with cinnamon, frankincense, lemon, and lavender.

Some oils can be inhaled. Add ten drops of appropriate oil in hot water or in a diffuser.

Some oils that can be safely applied directly to skin can also be used in direct palm inhalation. Apply one to two drops in palm. Rub hands together gently and inhale.

Oils can be added to bath. Mix lavender, frankincense, sandalwood, eucalyptus, or Texas cedarwood with milk, salts, or sesame oil so that it dispenses in water.

Oils can be used as a compress. Add ten drops in four ounces hot water, soak cloth, and wrap sore muscles.

Oils can be used in a facial steam. Add five drops of appropriate oil in a pot of hot water. Cover head with towel and steam. Excellent for opening sinuses and helping headaches when using appropriate oils.

Oils can be used in massage therapy. Add fifteen drops essential oil to one ounce carrier oil.

Many essential oils are strong enough to irritate the skin; therefore, carrier oils are used to dilute them and "carry" the oils onto our skin. Carrier oils also have therapeutic qualities.

PERSONALIZED HAIR AND SKIN CARE

We use simple and natural products for hair and body care, including:

Argan oil, jojoba oil, maracuja oil, sweet almond oil, and Jamaican Black castor oil.

Organic olive, avocado, coconut, and sesame oils are wonderful oils I use for cooking, skin and hair care, and oral hygiene.

I also blend shea, coconut, and mango butters with many of these carrier and essential oils for healthy and soothing body creams, deodorant, and hair conditioners.

There is a wealth of online information and recipes incorporating these products.

Facial

1 teaspoon avocado

1 teaspoon honey

1-2 teaspoons Braggs apple cider vinegar

1 teaspoon bentonite clay (DO NOT use metal bowls or utensils with clay. May destroy health properties.)

Mix into a paste and apply to face. Leave on for twenty minutes. Rinse with water and finish with equal parts Braggs apple cider vinegar and water. Tone with fresh slice of aloe vera. Moisturize with shea or cocoa butter.

Facial for Acne

1 teaspoon bentonite clay (Do Not Use Metal with clay)

Three drops each, lemon oil, lavender oil, and helichrysum oil.

1 teaspoon water

Mix into a paste and apply to face. Leave on for twenty minutes. Rinse; finish with equal parts Braggs apple cider vinegar and water. Tone with fresh slice of aloe vera.

Daily Facial Moisturizer and Skin Tightener

1/4 cup each, organic olive, coconut, and avocado oils

6 drops each, helichrysum oil, sandalwood oil, and cedar wood oil.

Store in a dark bottle.

Daily Facial Cream

1/2 cup raw cocoa butter

1/2 cup raw shea butter

1/4 cup blended Abba's oil and coconut oil

6 drops each, frankincense oil, sandalwood oil, and helichrysum oil

Melt cocoa butter over low heat. Add shea butter and melt. Remove from heat and let cool. Stir in oils.

Before Shampoo Hair Conditioner

Blend

1 tablespoon each, organic olive, coconut, and avocado oils, Jamaican Black castor oil

1 tablespoon each, melted shea butter, cocoa butter.

Apply a small amount to hair daily.

After Shampoo Hair Conditioner

Blend

1/4 cup organic mayonnaise

1/2 avocado

1 tablespoon coconut oil

1/4 -1/2 cup vodka

Wash hair and rinse. Apply conditioner and warm under shower cap for twenty minutes.

Remove cap and rinse.

Deodorant (DO NOT mix in or with metal containers or utensils if using clay)
1 tablespoon melted cocoa butter
1 tablespoon melted shea butter
1 tablespoon organic cornstarch
1 tablespoon dead sea salt, powdered
2 teaspoons bentonite or red clay, optional
Coconut oil, enough to make paste
3 drops each, tea tree oil, lemon oil, lavender oil, and eucalyptus oil.

Toothpaste
5 tablespoons organic coconut oil
1 tablespoon Himalayan pink sea salt, powdered
1 tablespoon trace minerals
2 tablespoons baking soda
3 drops organic myrrh essential oil
3 drops organic peppermint oil

Mouthwash
2 cups distilled water
1/2 cup Braggs apple cider vinegar
10 drops liquid trace minerals
5 drops each, cinnamon oil, clove oil, eucalyptus oil, helichrysum oil, myrrh oil, peppermint oil, and tea tree oil.

Gum Rinse #1

4 ounces water

2 drops each, hyssop oil, and Texas cedarwood oil

Add oils to water, swish, and expel. Do Not Swallow.

Gum Rinse #2

4 ounces water

2 teaspoons Himalayan sea salt

1/2 teaspoon Dead sea salt

20 drops calendula tincture

20 drops myrrh tincture or essential oil

Mix, swish, and expel. Do Not Swallow.

Skin Spritz

1 cup organic vodka

1/2 cup filtered water

10-20 drops of lavender, lemon, or ylang ylang oil. Mix together and store in a glass spray bottle.

Cuts and Scrapes

Organic Vodka

Tea Tree Oil

Helichrysum Oil

Either solution works well against bacteria.

Headache Remedy

Two drops each, clove oil, peppermint oil, eucalyptus oil, lavender oil, helichrysum oil, and cinnamon oil.

Mix essential oils in four ounces of olive oil or sesame oil and use to massage temples and shoulders. Store in a dark bottle.

Also, drink plenty of water to hydrate and detoxify. A pinch of Himalayan sea salt may also be added to an eight-ounce cup of warm water to drink.

CLEANING PRODUCTS WE USE

Our main household cleaner has been bottom-shelf rock-gut vodka. It has also served as an excellent bug killer and works well with white vinegar, baking soda, and different essential oils, depending on what it's needed for.

Kitchen Cleaner
Vodka
White vinegar
Biodegradable dish detergent
Tea tree oil
Pour a small amount of each ingredient on countertops and scrub. Rinse with water. For daily maintenance of cabinets and floors, omit detergent.

Add vodka, white vinegar, and lemon essential oil to detergent water to clean dishes, to add sparkle to glasses, and to clean sink fixtures.

Sprinkle baking soda on a cutting board surface and let sit for five minutes. Rinse with vodka, vinegar, and orange essential oil solution. Finish with clear water rinse.

If food gets stuck on the bottom of stainless steel pots and pans, cover the bottom with baking soda. Add a small amount of dish detergent and hot water. Bring to a boil; then, remove from stove and let sit to loosen food. Wash and rinse.

Bathroom Cleaner

Sprinkle baking soda in bathtub, sink, and toilet. Let sit approximately five to ten minutes. Pour a few drops of environmentally friendly dish or laundry detergent in each and scrub. Then pour in vodka and vinegar for final scrub. Rinse.

Vodka and vinegar solution will also clean and disinfect bathroom fixtures, walls, and floors.

Bathroom/Room Freshener

8 ounces vodka

2 ounces water

20 drops lemon oil, tea tree oil, lavender oil, or cinnamon oil. Experiment with another preferred oil or combination. Pour into a spray bottle.

For Smelly Clothes

If clothes are clean, but have underarm odor, saturate the area with pure vodka and hang to dry.

WHAT WE LEARNED ABOUT PLASTICS

Plastic #1 - Polyethylene Teraphalate (PET or PETE) Supposedly okay and is used for making water bottles, but good for single usage only.

Plastic #2 - High Density Polyethylene (HDPE) Also supposedly good to use. Used in making milk containers, grocery bags, trash and retail bags.

Plastic #3 - Polyvinyl Chloride (PVC) - BAD - It is thought that traces of this suspected human carcinogen is found in cling wrap plastics that wrap meats and cheeses, as well as in bibs, mattress covers, and shower curtains.

Plastic #4 - Low Density Polyethylene (PDPE) Supposedly okay. Used to wrap bread, make frozen food bags, squeezable bottles, plastic wrap (different from cling wrap), grocery store bags, and dry cleaning bags.

Plastic #5 - Polypropylene (PP) Supposedly okay, although it can be hazardous during the production of some ketchup bottles and yogurt tubs. It is not known to leach chemicals suspected of causing cancer.

Plastic #6 - Polystyrene (PS) - BAD - Benzene, a material used in production, is a known carcinogen. Butadiene and styrene are also suspected carcinogens. They are used for foam insulation and for hard substances, such as styrofoam cups, toys, opaque plastic spoons and forks, and meat trays.

Plastic #7 - Usually polycarbonate - BAD - Made with BPA. Supposedly used in the production of baby bottles, microwave ovenware, and eating utensils.

RETREAT AND REPRIEVE

Trials can be long and strenuous; so an occasional retreat is in order. Be refreshed and Live In Full Expectation.

LAUGH, LAUGH, LAUGH!!! We watch comedies when we need a good laugh, even if they're stupid.

COMMUNICATE! COMMUNICATE! COMMUNICATE! It's important to encourage Euvon to regularly discuss his thoughts and feelings about his diagnosis without him feeling self conscious. It's comparable to women confronting breast or vaginal cancer.

Cancer doesn't seem to do well in warm, fuzzy conditions; therefore, Euvon will **TAKE HOT SHOWERS,** sometimes twice a day, to soothe his bones and suffocate the adversary.

I often **RELAX IN A WARM BATH** filled with at least a cup of dead sea salts and a couple tablespoons of organic olive or avocado oil mixed with few drops of lavender, rose, and/or ylang ylang oil, depending on my mood. Then I listen to my favorite music or an online Bible study.

EXERCISE, EXERCISE, EXERCISE! Low impact or functional exercises have been included in our daily life, such as lifting low-pound weights, stationary biking, pilates, yoga, walking, or cleaning house.

DANCE, DANCE, DANCE!!! We dance as often as we can. One Valentine's Day during Euvon's immunotherapy, instead of our traditional dining out, we played music while preparing an organic meal together. Then we dined and danced the night away.

We **CHEAT!** At least twice a month we treat ourselves to one of those former cravings that haunts us still, such as a piece of fried chicken or a small piece of cake. Then we **PRAY, PRAY, PRAY** any toxins away.

We set aside some quiet time to **MEDITATE ON GOD'S WORD** and to **DEVELOP OUR FAITH**, which is the substance of things hoped for, the evidence of things not seen.

LOVE, LOVE, LOVE!!! Love yourself, love others, and love GOD, Who is our LIFE!

WHAT TO DO

So, what should someone do who has been diagnosed with a debilitating condition? PRAY, RESEARCH, PRAY, RESEARCH! If you can't do it, find someone who can. It was critically important for us to know everything we could about prostate cancer and how to precipitate Euvon's healing, regardless of its stage.

If insurance coverage is subpar, then go to some organization or somewhere to see if there are any available grants, take advantage of social media, and if that doesn't work, go on television and let the world cry for you also.

The woman in Mark's Gospel, who had the issue of blood for twelve years and touched Jesus's garment didn't have the media or a major news channel on her side. She just got out there in front of everybody, grabbed the hem of the Master's robe, and was healed. (Mark 5:25-34)

So, go somewhere you can be seen. Make yourself known. Tell your story. If you want to live, get loud in the marketplace.

A group of people tried to shut up the blind guy who, when he realized Jesus was walking by, screamed and hollered for help because he had nothing to lose. Yeshua heard him and he was healed. (Luke 18:35-43)

If you're about to go down, you'd better do something. Find a way.

Finally, GET YOUR REGULAR CHECKUPS!!!

For God so loved the world that He gave His only begotten Son, that whosoever believes in Him will not perish, but have everlasting life.

John 3:16

SELAH

"For dust you are, and to dust you will return." (Genesis 3:19); "We must die." (2 Sam.14:14); "A time to be born and a time to die." (Ecclesiastes 3:2); "We are confident...to be away from the body, and at home with the Lord." (2 Corinthians. 5:8).

Sit back, sip a cup of tea, and reflect on where you're going after death. Euvon and I realized from the beginning that regardless of how we lived, one day we are going to die because God said so. Our bodies will go to the grave, but our spirits will live on.

Our desire has been to live healthy and in obedience to the Lord. We've been muck-ups along the way, but His grace has been sufficient for us, His mercy has endured in our lives, and His lovingkindness has been directed toward us. And when we have finished this course, we will see Him in His glory.

Oh, we would that everyone loved the Lord because there are some things in life we can't bear on our own, and He never intended us to. He has always desired that men would call upon Him in love.

The Lord has been our Rock and our Salvation. He has been our Almighty God, our Counselor, our Abba, Father, our Prince of Peace, and we love Him. Our spirit man has been redeemed and sealed in Him by the Blood of Yeshua, Jesus, our Messiah, our Savior.

If church is not an option for Bible study, there are many online and printed Bible studies, as well as commentaries. So, take a peek into His Last Will and Testament, His Word, and pray that He will reveal Himself to you in a way that will provoke you to fall in love with Him and accept His Son, Yeshua, Jesus, as your Lord, Savior, and new best Friend. Amen.

For speaking engagements contact
Euvon Jones
e.byronassociatesinc@yahoo.com

The Trial of Stage IV Prostate Cancer

The Trial of Stage IV Prostate Cancer

www.ingramcontent.com/pod-product-compliance
Lightning Source LLC
Chambersburg PA
CBHW021856020426
42334CB00013B/362
* 9 7 8 0 9 9 0 9 6 2 6 0 1 *